FIONA PATRICE, MARCUS VALENTINE & CARLOS C.

SEX SEX SEX

J'aime le sexe

Taboo, Anecdotes, Tips, Advice and more.
Both sexes.

While every precaution has been taken in the preparation of this book, the publisher assumes no responsibility for errors or omissions, or for damages resulting from the use of the information contained herein.

SEX SEX SEX J'AIME LE SEXE

First edition. November 23, 2022.

Copyright © 2022 CARLOS C et al..

ISBN: 979-8215768990

Written by CARLOS C et al..

Table of Contents

Content:

- The Importance of Female Clitoral Orgasm
- The History Of Pay Per View Demand
- The French Kiss
- The Evolution From Video Cassettes To Adult Movies On Demand
- The Bonus to Confidence Given by Penis Enlargement is Priceless
- The Amazing Range Of Sex Toys
- The adventure of a Writer
- Status of Women in the Bible
- Spice Up Sex Life With Increased Ejaculation Volume
- Some Important Facts about Vibrators
- Size Matters More to Men

A BIG education

What is it with men and big boobs? Anatomically, these are glands which we humans use to feed our young. Technically its just another one of natures many designs to help us propagate and survive. As one may already know, breasts develop in the puberty stage with a girls hormones going haywire, no one can say how big its going to get. Studies say that the size of the breast depends on the support it gets from the chest. Breast growth increases rapidly during pregnancy and typically, the size of the breast fluctuates throughout the menstrual cycle. During old age, the breasts sag because the ligaments supporting it usually elongates.

Anyway, humans are the only animals in the kingdom animalia which has breasts that are permanently swollen, even when not lactating. Because of this, several studies have been made to find out the other functions of the breasts, more commonly known in the streets as big tit. According to scientists, animals mate when their partners are ovulating. Most animals know this because of the swollen breast of the female. For humans, this is also the same. Males find women with big boobs more attractive because it is associated with ovulation. Now for other primates, they usually have rear-entry copulation, thereby the basis for attractiveness is usually the buttocks. I know, rear-entry can also be done by humans, but of course, this wouldnt get the woman pregnant. Since sex is a basic instinct created by nature to propagate our species, we need to reproduce. It is said that the breast is the frontal counterpart of the buttocks, and due to our upright posture, humans are more likely to copulate face to face, or the position we know as missionary. This meant that because sex needed a face on encounter, the partners needed to develop a relationship which goes beyond the sexual one. Now of course these are the rantings of a woman whose breast size has always been smaller than the average.

In 1986, the dream of many boob-men in the world came true with the publication of Juggs, a softcore pornography magazine. The magazines name was actually the slang term for breasts. The magazine is still being printed today but there are other alternatives that replaced it in our modern world. You have big movie, and big tit porn. You have bouncing tits, big tit Latinas and big tit teens.

Unfortunately, despite the fascination of men in the US for big boobs, there are some cultures which dont think that it is a worthy area of study. Breasts were seen as natural as writers and painters refer to it time and time again without any qualms on the subject. According to studies, however, not all men, prefer big tits, the best size is always described as small, white, round like apples, hard, firm and wide apart.

7 Sex Tips for Parents

Sex life? What sex life? Youre a parent and life is so busy that you barely have time to think about your own needs, let alone do anything about meeting them. It can seem like your own needs dont matter, its the children that have top priority and you have to do whatever it takes to look after them. Dont be fooled, your needs are important and neglecting them isnt good for anyone, not you, not your partner and definitely not your children. Sure you cant do all the things you did before children, life has changed and pleasure comes in different ways. But you are still an adult with adult needs and for you to feel fulfilled they need to be met.

So how do you find time and energy for sex when there are so many other things demanding your attention? It takes a bit more planning and effort than in the past but you need to tell yourself that it can happen and it is definitely worth it.

What if you dont want anyone touching you after having children crawling all over you all day? Some people have a quotient for the amount of physical contact they need and can comfortably accommodate in a day. But if you think about it children touch you differently to how your partner touches you and for the most part, its all take.

So how do you have more sex? Okay, how do you have any sex?

1. Make it a priority and it will happen. Feeding the children quickly becomes a priority when you have nagging children at your feet. Make your desires like that and dont let up until you have got what you need.

2. Find a time that works. It may be early in the morning before the children wake up, it may be immediately after theyve gone to bed ignoring the dishes and the washing and cleaning up, it may be during the day while the kids are watching a video. You have to make time for each other.

3. Do some things that make you think about sex. It can be hard to switch your brain from babyland to sex so you may need a little help. Watch a sexy movie, read erotic fiction together, write your partner a sexy note, think back to a time when you had great sex (cmon you can do that, it cant be that long, surely, you have children afterall!), relive how good it felt.

4. Take a shower together. There is something about getting naked and wet together that can be very erotic.

5. Expect interruptions and dont be put off. OK you start kissing and you hear a baby cry. You try to ignore it but you cant. So you go off and tend to them and then think the moment is gone. But it isnt. And if it is then get it back by viewing the interruption as a diversion which has increased your appetite for sex not soured it.

6. Dont wait until you get into bed to initiate sex. When youve been together awhile its easy to fall into habits, like falling into a deep sleep as soon as your head touches the pillow, and sometimes its those habits that you need to break in order to kickstart your sex life. Sex can happen anywhere so make use of the spaces you have.

7. And the most important thing you need to do dont give up! You can find a way to make it happen. Know that your needs are important and you will function better when theyve been met.

3d sex games

They can also come in the form of variation of conventional online games such as card games with a sexual twist. There are multiplayer games or games that can be played with a computer generated character. It can be in a controlled setting with a theme or a very open-ended type game. There is something for everyone as games are made for persons of various sexual orientations, even bisexuals. No matter the type of game, there is fun to be had by adults using online sex games.

3d sex games are available with varied levels of interaction. They can be as as you want or can be require very little input from the player, consisting more of video-type content. Virtual characters can be personalized and selecting what they look like and wear, the types of activities they engage in, what they say or the situations they find themselves in. 3d sex games can also involve actual interaction with real persons versus playing against the computer. This can involves typed interaction or actual spoken and visual interaction using microphones and webcams. It is the new way to meet and date persons while attaining the optional, additional benefits. Men can enjoy instantaneous sex if they want and women can take it slower if thats what they wish to do, vice versa.

Some games allow you to access and update your virtual avatar in the online adult game on a continuous basis. 3d sex games can be testing grounds for the real world. Although online adult games in no way replace other social mediums persons may use these interactions to build confidence or to compensate for temporary periods of loneliness. The realm of online sex games is so varied that there is something to suit every type of individual or need. The number of games and features keeps growing to satisfy the wishes of gamers worldwide.

Playing a 3d sex game does not indicate that one is sex deprived or a sex freak. The simulations are so real that cybersex is becoming more and more attractive. In some cases it is simply used to spice up or complement an active sex life. These games can be used as a facilitator for cybersex among couples in a long distance relationship, for example. It can also be used as a medium through which fantasies that they are too shy to enact in real life can be acted out via the internet. It can be a couple's activity used to bring the two together in an intimate way. On the other hand, it can also be an anonymous and discreet way for persons to interact sexually with strangers, or new acquaintances. 3d sex games are made for adults to enjoy with each other can are very different from childish games. The aim is for the participants to have fun in an adult way, responsible but exciting way.

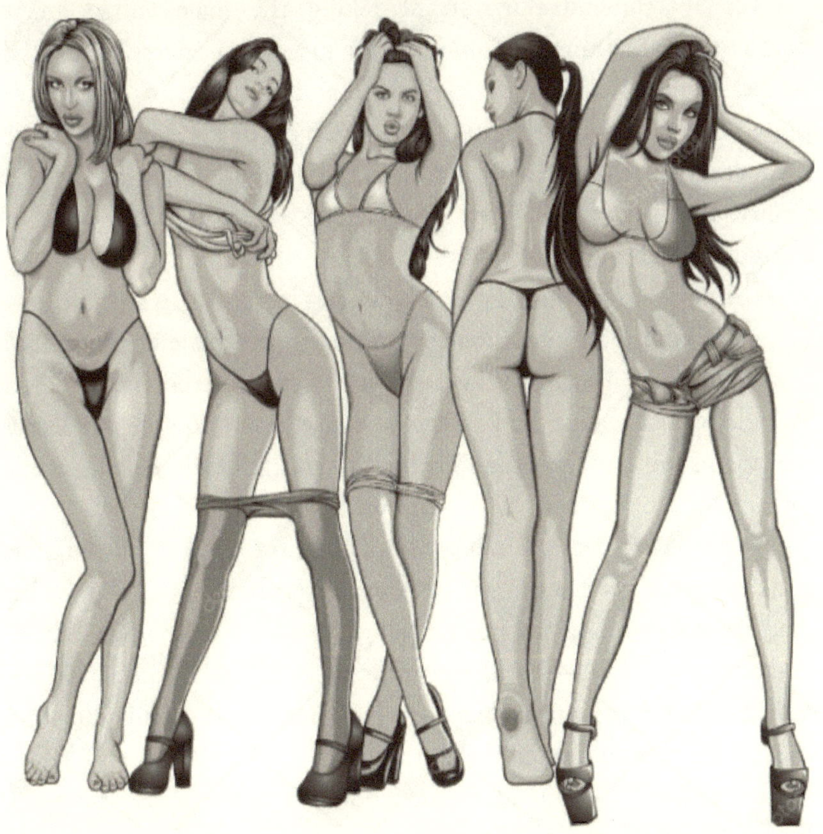

Your New Year Resolution : Make It Big And Strong

Your New Year Resolution : Make It Big And Strong

A growing number of men are turning to testosterone supplements to maintain energy levels as they age. The male enhancement supplements can be synthetic or herbal. It contains the perfect blend of potent ingredients to help increase the blood flow to the penis.

The recommend duration of taking the male enhancement supplements is minimum 3 months for maximum effectiveness. The Natural Male Enhancement supplements and formulated products give the additional benefits because of the natural ingredients which are used, and these ingredients play a dual role in improving sexuality and virility. They share some of the same benefits of Viagra, but they are in a league of their own.

The popularity of these pharmaceuticals has spawned a whole new line of natural male enhancement products. Our male enhancement supplements are designed using a specific blend of herbal nutritents to provide optimal blood flow to the genital region. However we know that penis pills when combined with natural penis enhancement techniques can significantly enhance your penis.

You will come across hundreds of websites offering information and even products that claim to help you to stay hard but do they really. And they are among the hottest-selling products in the $26 billion herbal supplement — or as the makers call them, nutraceutical — industry. In the meantime, men who have heart disease and are taking cardiac drugs should avoid these products.

Because our pills provides more blood flow to the penis, your penis 'hangs' larger all day. If you're like most men, you've probably already tried one or many of the penis enlargement pills and patches on the market today. The ingredients in the Natural Gain Plus Enhancement pills are taken from nature, and these assure that you can increase the size, volume and thereby the much talked about sexual pleasure. Join thousands of satisfied customers and experience for yourself the proven benefits of Natural Gain Plus.

For a number of reasons, men can experience a decrease in natural blood flow during arousal that can lead to difficulties in getting and maintaining erections. Most men have complaints related to sexual satisfaction (a desire for longer-lasting erections or more stamina, for example) versus a physical dysfunction like premature ejaculation or the inability to get an erection and maintain it for his partner's sexual pleasure. I used to not last very long and my erections were not very hard, but with this product I last longer and please the woman I'm with (which increases my confidence). My erections are much, much harder and also much thicker.

Male enhancement supplements work increase the amount of blood flow the genital region receives and the volume of blood that it can retain. Natural Gain Plus is the most powerful natural male enhancement pill available anywhere in the world. It is made from all natural products and the product site does not report any side effects from taking Natural Gain Plus.

Natural Gain Plus is specially formulated just for men, and contains a special blend of nutrients that can stimulate circulation to the penis as well as balance the body's natural hormones and relax the mind. Maca is considered by top researchers to be a true adaptogen. Maca is consumed as food for humans and livestock, suggesting any risk from consumption is rather minimal.I asked Antonio if he used these plants himself. He smiled again. "Sometimes. After all, I've been married to the same woman for 43 years."

You Might Find The Girl Next Door; Live On Web

You Might Find The Girl Next Door; Live On Web cam, Waiting For You

Today most of the people enjoy the opportunity to have some fun with the hot and adult woman with web cams on the Internet. Various known chat rooms are available now to fulfill our most wanted desires. There are mature sexy woman who are usually ready to chat with anyone at any topic hours after hours with no hesitance and tiredness. The hot woman with web cams generally starts with hot discussions and then shows off their physical beauties through web cams live as one visitor ask them while chatting. These cam sexy womens hides nothing and are quite frank. They are always there to do anything to satisfy the needs and desires of their visitors in the chat rooms. Actually precisely speaking these adult webcam girls on adult chat rooms is only to provide pleasure to us as much as possible. The hot women with adult webcams are always anxious and ready to fulfill our fantasies any time at the cost of something which often they asks to the visitors.

These adult sexy women share everything with us, and talk about the innermost feelings and thoughts. They usually try to understand our feelings for them and they reacts accordingly enabling us to hear and also see them through the web cam. Actually they do not mind at all and usually they are quite free and not at all shaky to chat with them at any topic in any manner. They also give reply to the visitors taking in mind to satisfy them most. The sexy womans in live adult webcams brings excitement and curiosity among the visitors to know everything about them including their physical structures. As time goes on chatting with anyone, the adult sexy womans gets ready to make some naughty actions. These sexy babes on web cam usually reveal on everything to the thousands or even more whoever comes to the adult chat rooms.

After chatting for a few hours with a cam girl, a special bondage usually forms within the visitors. The sexy women reveal almost everything to entertain and provide pleasure continuously by any means.

If our partner too wants to join and experience the exciting moments with the cam girls, they are also permitted to this. Actually one feels much better along with a partner in enjoying the hottest chats with the hot and sexy cam girls all together. The adult webcam girls are the only one who can provide the correct inspiration for the couples to try out new procedures of having sex. The sexy girls on web cam usually boost our curiosity towards sex in the correct procedures.

There are so many hot and sexy adult webcam girls available through out the web. One has the right to choose in accordance to their personal choice knowing their look and physical structures by going through their profile before hand of chatting. It takes only a single click of a mouse to share our feelings to them. The hot cam girls being experienced, they would help to us to become crazy that one would remember for a long time.

Would you like to be known as a sex god

Would you like to be known as a sex god ?

The most common problem for couples looking for better sex is that they don't look outside of their comfort zone. More sex is not better; better sex is better; for the tangoe-ing twosome and humankind as a whole. Better sex is the essence of better health. In many cases, people seem to think the way to achieve better sex is simply to have less bad sex.

Women notice if a man is confident in his abilities, and will want to get to know him better. Women are very adept at reading a man, and this is one area that they will want to be sure of before approaching the man. Women report that they prefer longer sexual sessions that include massaging, masturbation and oral sex stimulation, as well as penetration. Women and Men spend millions of amount on drugs and medicines annually for increased Sex Power & Sex Time.

Sexual Ability All women expect a man to know how to please them. Sexual satisfaction has always been important to us, and it should be something we keep achieving throughout our lives. All the same, for those who feel sexually bored or inadequate and are far from confident that they know all there is to know, the better sex guides are not to be sneered at. Its a great way to develop a more subtle and varied sexual repertoire and to discover new dimensions of erotic pleasure. It offers a very practical and scientific approach to improving the reader's sexual health.

Expand your sexual repertoire and discover how toys can stimulate your senses, excite your desires and fulfill your fantasies. It's not just the immense cultural pressure to be good at sex, and the fact that society has become very sexualised, it's that sex doesn't always come naturally. Similarly women can become more sexually responsive, more orgasmic, increase their potential to experience G spot orgasm and maintain urogenital health as they get older. The benefits of engaging in regular sexual intercourse include weight loss, stress reduction, improved circulation and increased longevity. Exercise done properly enhances sexual functioning because it can naturally increase testosterone levels in both males and females.The message is that we all need to wake up about our sexual health, start managing it more effectively, and encourage our friends to do the same regardless of our sexuality.

Online sex guides are a good choice because they have videos and pictures and can be accessed from anywhere. We believe Lovecentria is the best online sex tutor available, click here to become a member in minutes. Enjoy more sex and better sex with our #1 sex guide Lovecentria is a new online sex guide which will turn you in to a much envied sexual expert.

Each technique that men and women need to know to become true experts in bringing sexual joy to their partners is set forth in explicit detail, and some are graphically and artistically illustrated by the author.

Will Sex Toys Help Make Men Indispensable?

The answer to this question lies in the biological and social roles of males and females and in the way that sex toys may replace the role of men in those relationships.

Simplifying the subject considerably, evolution has resulted in most species having males and females for sexual reproduction resulting in the sharing and diversification of the gentic pool. However the existence of two 'versions' of a species has also allowed the development of specialisations/roles for the males and females.

In mammals the main biological difference is that the male provides sperm and the female provides eggs. After fertilisation the female has the role of looking after the embryo in the uterus (womb) and providing milk to the offspring after birth.

With this simple view the male provides only the sperm and a widening of the gene pool. However it would generally be too expensive in resources (in evolutionary terms) for that to be the only role of males, and so social responsibilities have evolved. Males often look after their mate and offspring by helping to provide food, protection and a 'home'.

With humans, changes in much of the world mean that many of these social roles can be provided by women alone and some women argue the world would be better off without men. Additionally biological advances may make men unnecessary for their biological role of fertilisation of the eggs.

The last remaining need for men might become one of providing entertainment and sexual satisfaction for women – but perhaps women could do without men for sex!

There is a growing move towards women turning to other women for sexual relationships; women are using sex toys more often as penis substitutes and many women find they get greater sexual satisfaction from sex toys (as measured by strength, frequency and reliability of orgasm) than they do from sex with men.

Some women act out the male role by using a strap-on harness and many dildos represent a man's penis. On the other hand many women prefer to exclude the male phallic image from their sexual play and they choose a vibrator or dildo that is not phallic and may indeed have a distinctly feminine design as does the Natural Contours Ultime vibrator.

This simple picture, though perhaps frightening for men, is rather too much of a simplification. Many women have a psychological need for men as a partner in life and sex (as men do for women). Probably for most women this will always be the case. These women usually also enjoy sex toys, using them both on their own and with their partners to get more satisfaction and enriching their relationship.

If women as a whole could choose whether men existed or not I feel sure they would come down on the side of keeping them. However if some other reason arose why men had become undesirable then women have already shown they could do without them quite easily ...

Why You Shouldn't Be Scared of Adult Toys

Remnants of the free love generation have thankfully survived and in recent years a sexual revival has resurged in the American psyche and bedroom. This time, however, the participants are a bit wiser and more sophisticated in their sexual exploration. As a result sex toys, once limited to the margins of society, have come full circle and are now in the mainstream of American living. Individuals and couples who had never before tried sex toys are now doing so for the first time. And yet, there still remains some who are scared of introducing sex toys into their life.

This fear comes in large part from a misunderstanding about the uses and ramifications of sex toys. They imagine that sex toys are limited to extreme versions of fetishism or that somehow sex toys are a means of separating you from your partner. These two conclusions cannot be farther from the truth.

With the recent explosion in the popular usage of sex toys, manufacturers have created a wide array of products designed to meet the needs and interests of everyone. While certainly there exists a wide array of S & M products on the market today which those interested in find extremely fun, there also exist a number of products designed for the novice user.

The sex toy industry is completely aware of the desire for many individuals to keep their toys discrete. As a result, a number of products have been designed with that end in mind. Vibrators that look exactly like lipstick containers and lotions and lubricants which are described with terms like relaxation rather than more explicit sexual terminology come to mind. The discrete design and packaging of sexual toys allows even the shyest of individuals to feel comfortable.

With fears allayed as to the nature of sex toys, the next question is about their effects on an existing relationship. Whereas in decades past sex toys were largely limited to single individuals or those focused on a particular area of sex, normally labeled fetishism, recently sex toys have been brought into millions of couples bedrooms. Sex toys can be a new and exciting way to spice up sex between a couple who has been together for some time. It can also be an excellent way for couples to explore new areas to find that something works better for them. In effect, sex toys, rather than creating division between couples, are often a source which brings them together in new and exciting romantic situations.

Why is ejaculation control for men so important?

Once a man has reached the point in his sexual development where he begins to understand that just "getting off" isn't satisfying him or his partner, he craves for more. Which is a natural desire. And in his heart he knows there is more, but often doesn't know how to achieve these higher pleasures. Tantra teaches us that for a man to achieve the highest Ecstasy possible for himself and his lover, he first needs to learn ejaculation control and to direct his sexual energy up his spine to the higher centers of his brain. In Tantra this sexual energy is known as "kundalini" energy.

When a man masters the ability to move his Kundalini energy up along his spine, he increases the pleasure for himself and his lover to levels that he might never have dreamt of. As a man learns to master the movement his Sexual Energy within his body, he will be able to control his ejaculation. At this point he is free to make love "without" feeling the pressure to ejaculate.

A man's sensitivity and awareness is profoundly heightened to the subtle and refined pleasures of lovemaking. He steps into an expanded state of consciousness, which allows him to achieve "multiple" and "full-body orgasms". The benefits of "full-body" orgasm are many. Full-body orgasm frees him from stress and tensions, heals his prostate gland, opens his heart and connects him deeper to his lover and himself. It also facilitates the man in experiencing multiple orgasms. By "multiple" is not to imply "multiple ejaculations", but rather that once a man learns to move his Kundalini energy through his body he can have orgasms and not ejaculate. This is known as a "dry orgasm" or none-ejaculatory orgasm.

Men have a tremendous capacity for pleasure and orgasm that is virtually untouched for most men. As a man masters tantric practice and higher energy movement, he begins to view his Lingam (penis) as an instrument of a deeper love connection with the woman. This deeper connection facilitates moving the woman to the highest states of Ecstasy and orgasmic pleasure that she can achieve. Allowing the man and woman to continue to build higher levels of ecstasy together.

Why buy adult films?

Feeling horny but no ones there to feed your fantasies? Tired of staring at those porn photos? Been wanting to see a real action? Despair no, adult dvds are here to the rescue! Feast your eyes with these hot babes who are just too willing to give you a peek on one of their so-loved body parts or on guys naughtily playing their shafts as they get harder and harder. Be amazed with how a chick would so enjoy being licked by three totally naked all around her body.

Share the feverish sensation with a couple screaming in pleasure while they both are about to reach the seventh heaven. Feel and enjoy how a woman on top position would make a guy crazy and would keep asking for more. It would not be a shame to admit if we do enjoy these movies. Well if it pleases you, then go for it. If you think that people watch porn films just because they are kinky, think again; there is more to than just gratifying themselves. There are some people who feel insecure in bed. They think that they are not a good bed partner, that they are not capable of giving their mates the best sack session or in other words they are boring bed mates.

Lovemaking is a physical manifestation of couples love for each other and of course as a mate it is a sort of obligation to give your partner the things that would make her happy and that include sex. Need a sex teacher who could give you the best sex techniques and be the best sex partner? Nope, you dont need to enroll in a sex crash course. All you have to do is buy porn dvds or do a porn dvd download. Xxx porn dvds are the best sex teachers you can easily rely on. Learn and master the techniques and you will be a sex guru or sex god in the making and maybe you can even write a sex book in the future. Good and helpful entertainment need not to be expensive, invest on cheap porn dvds and learn the know-how in bringing your mate to the seventh heaven. But remember not all people who keep adult dvds do have the same purpose.

Some are just curious or a few might just want to come up with a good term paper about porn films. Whatever the reason is,always remember to be responsible viewers or owners of these materials. No one could stop us from watching titillating movies but it would not hurt us to be a little careful. Watch them with the right people of the right age at he right places of course. So what are you waiting for, do not deprive yourselves of the things that would give you happiness and satisfaction. They say do what pleases you so there would be no reason for you to stop yourself from enjoying these movies. Porn dvds might just be the answer to your sex problems.

Why Am I Not Interested In Sex?

There is a frightening trend going on in many of the marriages and serious relationships of today — no sex. I know you've heard all the clichs. Especially the one about couples not having sex after they get married. But really...what they should say is that the sex can truly diminish after having children and being consumed with the stressors of raising them, feeding them, and schooling them!

I mean who really has the energy or the gumption to look sexy, feel sexy, and better yet have sex! Children are a lot of work. Hey, life is a lot of work. Is this why our mothers were so irritable when we were little?

Well, if you want to live in reality – eventually you have to address this lack-of-sex subject in your marriage. Married folks have sex, and should enjoy it, and hopefully desire it on at least a semi-regular basis. We need it.

So why are so many of us not handling this subject like we would our finances, our careers, our children? Why are we avoiding it? Well, because even in todays modern society, sex is still a very uncomfortable subject for us to discuss with our children, our friends, and our spouses.

Its strange isnt it? We love a good romance novel, or romantic comedy movie. So why arent we talking? Well, in many cases we feel that we are the source of the problem, but we are confused or frightened to admit it and deal with it.

If this sounds like you and your marriage there may be a few concrete ways you can address what has to be a very difficult and painful topic for you and your spouse. Lets get back to intimacy.

First – if you have a diminished desire for sex, go see your physician and check yourself out. Hormone levels fluctuate. Having children can throw you out of wack. Make sure it isn't a physical problem.

Also, there are some women who have always experienced uncomfortable or even painful sex during intercourse but never addressed it. Perhaps you think that certain positions are just not meant for you, but it may be that you have a physical problem that has a solution. Simply stated – if you can't get aroused or are uncomfortable, even after a round of foreplay, there may be something physical going on. Check it out with your gynecologist.

Second – If you check out okay, and there is nothing physically wrong with your partner, then you can assume that the problem is probably something mental/emotional in nature.

Are you tired? Mentally tired? Tired of him? Is he still attractive to you or is he just a warm body? Do you feel unattractive? Do you think he feels you are unattractive? Have either of you cheated in the past – and know about it? Is sex boring–A ritualistic rut?

It's a huge myth that sex is not an important part of a relationship. Physical intimacy with your partner is very important for the health of your relationship.

If you are dating, you SHOULD be sexually attracted to the person. If you are not, you may face serious problems in the future.

If you are married, sex may not feel like it did the first time with him, but it should be satisfying and desired by both of you. Low feelings of desire?

1. Pinpoint your sources of stress. Write them down. Number them. Get a list. What is causing you the most stress? Finances? Intimacy? Children? Illness? Family?

2. Now sort them in their order of importance. The last item on the list you should be able to eliminate this week. For example, if your kids are stressing you out. Hire a babysitter; go out on a date with your mate, and at the end of the evening try to initiate intimacy.

3. Continue to work on whittling down your list while you keep up with your

date nights etc.

4. Find things to reduce your overall stress levels. Activities such as reading a book, yoga, walking/running, taking up an old hobby, dancing to your favorite music on your Ipod, etc.

Reducing your overall stress is a great way to promote relaxation during times of intimacy. Sometimes we put great amounts of performance pressure on ourselves and inadvertently sabotage our performance. Plus happy people have more sex! Well, Im not sure about that statistically but it makes sense right?

What is porn for?

Ever tried watching live sex feed on the internet? How about live teen cam? Sure you can say no but you see a lot of people watch live porn cam not to get turned on but to pass the time. Let me give you an illustration.

Last night, I asked one of my male friends how do you make a review of something you have no idea about? This is not to say that I never watched porn before, but as a matter of fact, the first time I was exposed to nude men and women was when I was in college. Anyway, back then, I was the only female in the room so I had to ask them to watch with the TV on mute because it was so noisy and I didnt want my landlady to hear the sound. I asked the question with one of the guy buddies I lived with before and the answer was pretty simple. He said: Well, why dont you watch it, with sound this time and see what you feel afterwards. He then advised me to share my experience through my review.

Fact is I have always avoided watching porn, especially when I am with my friends. Truthfully, I feel uncomfortable because I dont know how I should react, whether I should just shut up or keep commenting. Anyway, I turned on my laptop and plugged in my headset (to make sure no one else can hear what I will hear), and started watching couples having sex on the web. After the feed, well, I still felt the same. I was expecting to get turned on or something, but the truth is, I wasnt not because I didnt like what I saw but probably because I had too many questions reeling on my mind.

So I sent an IM to my friend and told him what happened. He laughed at me and said: Well, did you think that porn is magic? Of course it can help get you in the mood but it isnt an alternative for the real thing. He also told me his opinion of porn: that it is raw and how sex should be. He said that most people are actually afraid to experiment so they end up faking their moans and still unsatisfied after coming. This is because they deny themselves the pleasure of enjoying the act. Well, truth is, Im starting to understand his point. Maybe porn is not as dirty as what most people think it is, maybe this is people are wanting to do but never had the courage to try with their partners because of their fear to be labeled crude, vulgar and uncouth.

Webcam action couldn't get hotter

There are millions of sites on the Internet that promise you a whale of a time with their version of sex shows on the web cam and web cam chats. You must have tried your luck with many of these sites but the desire seems to be ever growing. Check out our site and experience a whole new world of sex chats and web cam chats. The models are hot and can make a hard man like you melt. They are the best and you will know why we say so, simply try out and feel the heat.

Web cam chats are pretty popular nowadays but its interesting if only the model on the other side can rouse you up. Our models can set you on fire. Try them and you will never try out another porn site. You simply let your desire loose. Web cam chats, sex shows on the web cam it is all hers. Enjoy and rejuvenate your sensual perceptions on the web cam while the models perform on you. Chat up with them over telephone and see the on the web cam performing whatever your desire commands. Its an experience that will blow your mind. Truly, the models will ignite your passion and set your obsession free. Choose from a range of sexy hot babes. American, Latin, Asian, and Oriental it is all here and they are waiting to satisfy your desires.

Dont miss the sex shows, they are performed by bombshell hotties and they are the best as you will see when you try them out. You lay a wager that you are going to have the most amazing time of your life. Get overwhelmed by the desire roaring within you and then you can call up and engage in a stimulating sex chat with the hot babes, while they perform sex acts on the web cam. The models are the best in the business and can perform any sex act on the web cam. You drop out your desire and their magic charm will satisfy your deepest desire. Go for it and feel the heat.

Thats not all. Check out and download directly from the amazing range of HD quality porn videos that are on the web site. There are no hidden costs and all the videos are of superior quality. Download and watch them in your free time and nurture your deepest and best kept secret desires.

Your deepest desires are very special and so the models take every bit of care to ensure that your satisfaction is guaranteed. This website does not aimlessly propose and deliver short of your desires, log in, try out and you will never again try out any other porn site on the internet.

Wake Up America sex toys are Sweeping the Nation

It's time to get busy, America. Sex toys are now out of the closet and on bedside tables everywhere, and this fun, steamy, fully illustrated website will walk you through the process of choosing, buying, and having a creative blast with your sex toys. Sex toys for women, sex toys for men, sex toys for both.

Couples and singles alike can enjoy sex-toy activities, laid out like recipes, and complete with tips for spicy variations. You will learn the male g spot, the female g spot, how to locate them. How to stimulate the g spot and sex toys to stimulate both Add vibrators to your favorite sex positions. Spice up your masturbation routine and toys for masturbation. Liven up oral sex with lubes and lotions and sex toys for oral sex.

Get comfortable with anal sex. Questions and answers from the most common questions, posted to alt sex binarys. Learn how to enjoy anal sex.

How to choose the proper sex toy for you. Complete with an explanation on textures and types available, the proper size that would be comfortable for you

With sex toy Web sites thriving and sex toy parties sweeping the nation (move over, Tupperware), This unique website provides a perfect dose of inspiration to get those toys fired up and ready to roll. Pictures complete with products details Fun sex education with illustrations.

Victoria Sin Redefines Dirty

The pornography industry is one that is consists of many genres, as producers and porno stars are looking to create an availability for dirty materials o matter what someones tastes or preferences. Besides so many websites and videos on demand and various pornographic outlets, the genre of filthy whore porn is popular for those guys really looking to get off hard from seeing a filthy slut take the dick in many different ways. Often times filthy whore porn is more graphic than other genres because after all, hookers, whore, prostitutes or sluts, no matter what you call them, are known for being sexually promiscuous. Scenes in these types of films often include many men at a time in gang bang orgy scenarios where a dirty whore is either sitting on a dick that is up her ass, taking another in her pussy and of course sucking on another or jerking some lucky man whore off. These dirty whore role play scenarios also are thematic with the names of the stars in the adult films. Victoria Sin is one such name that would ring a bell among those fans of dirty whore porn and similarly filthy videos and imagery aimed to make horny men cum hard.

Victoria Sin is an example of a porno name that might include an element of the actress actual name, maybe her first name is Victoria or last name Sin, maybe not both. Whatever the case, it is sinful not to want to watch as hot horny women depicted as hustling prostitutes get laid in a variety of positions and of course showing off their flexibility and acrobatic skills. Besides porn, men are often times interested in moves commonly related to whoring, such as a woman pulling her legs behind her head, taking a hard, long cock in the ass and one in the vagina at the same time. These types of relations usually do not occur in real life, that is why dirty whore porn is popular where men and their fantasies, and of course gays can be equally as interested in this type of pornographic material as well.

Victoria Sin may be an adult film star within the super dirty, filthy, but hot and sexy world of hooker porn and gang bang type scenarios, but nonetheless, this porn and every type of porn for that matter is for men and women eighteen years and up to enjoy and perhaps even masturbate to, never under any circumstance can minors obtain these materials due to a companys negligence and if they do then that is a punishable crime in most states.

Vaginas and Oral Simulators

Vagina is a simulator of female genitals sometimes equipped with vibrator or pomp.

Oral Simulator is a sex toy imitating mouth and creating the oral sex effect. By its functional features oral simulator is similar to vagina.

Nowadays *sex shops sell sex toys* with vibrating and sucking functions; therere also simple self-driven toys, non-visual-effect toys and toys imitating all female genital details: vulvar lips, anus or pubic hair.

Man experiences real bright sensations while using vagina, since the penis is actively massaged by vaginal walls. Moreover, if vagina is equipped with soft knobbles or ribs and vibrating or sucking mechanism, the man gets incomparable orgasm.

Vaginas and oral simulators create double effect: first diversity in sexual life, second physical and psychological unload of organism. Both men and women may have psychological disorders as well as overstrain or alcohol overconsumption problems, which may cause temporary asthenia or even importance. Importance also depends on prostate condition -approximately 40% of men after 40 suffer from prostatitis. And again artificial vagina will be of great help here.

Vagina or oral simulator can be used independently and with a partner to enhance erection. Vagina is also important for prevention of congestions, prostatitis and adenoma. Pelvis and genitals blood congestion result in male genital system inflammations and diseases. To avoid such congestions, men before 40 should ejaculate 2-3 times a week, and after 40 no less than once a week. However therere situations when theres no woman about: military service, business trip etc. Afterwards long continence may cause poor erection or quick ejaculation, with a man getting strong psychological shock and, as a result, importance. Artificial vaginas can solve all these problems.

Modern **sex shops offer a good deal of vaginas, anuses and oral simulators** of all possible modifications made of latex, silicone, cyber-skin etc. They all make up for a woman absence, diversify sexual relations and add them some special shading.

Realistic vaginas are very useful for sexual upbringing of your teen son. They can be used to learn female genitals structure and for practice. At 13-14 real sex with real woman wont always be good but vice versa can result in psychological injuries. At this age a boy turns into a man and masturbation is inevitable, i.e., the best way out is artificial vagina. Its usage will provide for the general hygiene of your childs genitals and protect him from all possible infections.

Use of Sex Toy Not Safe While Driving

Have you seen the ad for the sex toy called Auto Suck? It goes like this:

"Enjoy your drive with the ideal mate! Plugs into any car or truck lighter for some hot roadway action. Make sure to keep one hand on the wheel and one eye on the road as the auto suck makes that long commute or road trip much more bearable. *Warning: this unit may cause ejaculation. This may be difficult to explain to your insurance company. Use at your own risk!".

Okay, Im not a prude and I know everyone is entitled to good sex, I understand its our right and Im all for it, but please....Is it really safe or necessary to use one of these units while driving? I think not! Look at the distraction problems we already face on the roads everyday. All the fancy billboards and roadside signs that flash or scroll. The idiots who just have to be on their cells phones while driving just to mention a few. Now, throw in a portable sex toy like the Auto Suck and Im scared to death to be out on the road!

Seriously, and answer honestly, how many of you can keep your eyes open when you are having an orgasm? Come on, its like sneezing, you just cant do it! So lets give this toy to the male driver and hope for the best. Yeah this is just what I want a guy to be doing while driving a huge 20,000 pound, 550 H/P, 13 speed/overdrive tractor trailer. Seat belts and air bags wont mean anything if you collide with one. Can you imagine the lawsuit implications with one of these toys? The ad actually suggests using it while driving. How stupid are they?

In my opinion your just asking for trouble if you use one of these while driving. If you want to wait until you get to a rest stop or someplace safe to pull off and then hook up with the Auto Suck, fine Ive got no complaints. To each their own. I suppose used safely it could be considered an "ideal mate". But I just don't understand what the advertisers of this toy were thinking.

In 2004, there were over 6 million motor vehicle crashes in the United States (data for 2005 is not yet available). The National Highway Traffic Safety Administration (NHTSA) reported a total of 38,253 fatal crashes. There were 42,636 fatalities in those crashes. Non-fatal crashes totalled a whopping 6,143,000 with over 2.7 million personal injuries reported. There was an additional 4.2 million crashes related to property damage.

Given these statistics and the numerous distractions that drivers face every-day I can only hope that if anyone purchases the Auto Suck toy, they have enough intelligence not use it while driving.

A New Way For Adult Webmasters To Start Their Own

A New Way For Adult Webmasters To Start There Own Site

Welcome to Ultimate-tgp Dynamic Tgp Affiliate Program!

Ultimate-tgp offers you a powerful Dynamic Tgp affiliate site with FREE HOSTING, Trade script , one click Sponsor adding ,Premade Templates, and 195758 Galleries And 338 Sponsors. and growing

We pay to every webmaster 70% of his/her subscriptions and re-bills. Webmasters who have more than 50 subscriptions per month, get 80% of their subscriptions and re-bills.

Join Ultimate-Tgp!

There is absolutely no cost to join! Just fill out the signup form and login to the members area using your member login and password provided on the registration page. We do review every application by hand to maintain the quality of our program and to assure our sponsors that we admit only serious adult webmasters. For this reason, there may be a short delay in processing your application.

Forward Your Domain To Your Member Address Using The Mask Or Hide Url Option.

Choose Your Template And Layout.

Log in and go to AffiliateTools Edit template Select a template of your choice and email us your logo (On New Templates We will Do The Logo).

Add Your Sponsors In The Members Area.

All new Ultimate-Tgp customers must promote our Sponsors with our approved Affiliate code(s), which represent the best of the best in the adult industry. Once you have finished the sign up process select as many sponsors as you can to get best results. You will gain access to our expanded database of over 200 affiliate programs to choose from. Of course, we only make our money if you are successful in promoting your site. Each sponsor has a different payout structure, But we payout on a weekly basis.

We Setup And Enter Your New Ultimate Sponsor Codes In Your Members Area Upon Activation.

Once you select your Sponsor(s) by clicking the appropriate link on the Affiliate Tools Page of the Member's Area, we do the rest.

Make Money!

We don't make money unless you make money! So we are truly your partner! We're here to help you be more successful. Take advantage of the Ultimate-Tgp community...Many of our users depend solely on Ultimate-Tgp to make a living. We challenge you to find a host, paid or otherwise, who offers as much as Ultimate-Tgp! It costs nothing to create an account...join us today!

Please note all free member accounts Affiliate url's are selected randomly But you do have to option to upgrade.

Ubersexuals: The New American Man?

Forget "metrosexuals." The hot new man in town is the "ubersexual."

That's right, just when you thought you finally understood the metrosexual trend, it turns out that the new uber male not only exudes confidence and leadership, but-and this may be the crucial difference-does it all while still embracing his masculinity. In other words, as one trend spotter recently put it, ubers mark "the return of 'The Real Man' of yesteryear."

So the burning question is: How else does an uber differ from a metrosexual?

Well, both groups have female friends; however, an ubersexual's best pals are males, while a metrosexual's are females.

Both ubers and metros may groom themselves with expensive products-in fact, nearly two out of three men recently surveyed said they own and consistently use a variety of grooming products. The difference is that you won't catch an ubersexual highlighting, waxing or self-tanning.

One thing ubers and metros do have in common is a love of pearly white teeth-and as far as ubers are concerned, the whiter, the better. In fact, one survey found that 70 percent of them think white teeth go hand in hand with great hairstyles when it comes to the top two most important facial features. Yet, three out of four ubers admit their teeth "could be whiter."

The same survey found that ubers had no qualms about strolling into a store to pick up a personal grooming product such as Crest Whitestrips Premium. To add an especially "uber-masculine" twist to the strips, men sometimes put them on for 30 minutes, twice a day, while watching sports on TV. They get a whiter smile in just three days, with full results in seven.

Women looking for just the right uber may want to take note of the survey, too. Nearly half of men stressed that white teeth are a deciding factor when asking a woman on a second date. Also, one in five men said they absolutely couldn't kiss someone with yellow teeth.

Touching A Man's Penis – The Right Way

As women, we are usually at a loss as to how to touch a mans penis in a way that is wonderfully pleasuring to him. Our man wants us to bring him to orgasm manually, but we have NO clue has to how to do that. How tightly do we hold his cock? How far up and down his shaft to we move our hands? How do we hold our hands on him as we stroke him?

Getting a man to experience orgasm as we touch him is often a lengthy process. We feel so clumsy about it, and we often ARE clumsy about it, that our arm wears out before he cums. Then in frustration he moves our hand aside and does it himself, right, the first time.

Now bear in mind, that every man does himself differently. They all have techniques that feel best to them. So you may have to experiment, ask questions (in a sexy tone) and watch how he does it himself. (A woman raptly watching him masturbate from close up is a real turn-on to a man). You may have to induce him to let you watch. Try offering to let him cum in your mouth or on your breasts as an inducement. Remember that as they get closer to cumming, they often change techniques. Watch for that. DONT ask questions when he is close to cumming. Gently playing with his testicles as you watch is a great way to help out. Men love to hear us squeel in delight as they start to shoot.

So, if you can get your man to show you how HE does it, you are miles ahead! But in general, for a starter, try these things. Well . . . here is how I do it for my lover.

1) Place your body where you can rest your wrist on his hip or tummy and still be able to move your hand an inch and a half or two inches by flexing your wrist back and forth. This will help with your fatigue factor. I usually lie on my mans right side, my shoulder about level with his, and I put my head on his shoulder or on the pillow beside his head. I use my right hand to stroke him. (I am right handed.)

2) Wrap your first finger and thumb around his cock shaft two inches below his glans (the cute little crown men have at the bottom of their little helmet). You will move your hand from that location up to just below his crown, but not over his crown. That is your stroking range. Readjust your position beside him so that you can move your hand up and down his cock this distance by simply flexing your wrist, your wrist and forearm resting on him. Remember, this may take awhile, so get comfy.

3) Stroke SLOW. Dont wear yourself out by doing it fast. Nice slow movements up and down his shaft are the key. You will feel his cock continue to harden if you are going the right speed. If his cock begins to soften, you are doing it wrong (Make your fantasy more lurid, slow your speed, let your little finger caress his balls each time you come to the bottom of your stroke).

4) Breathe in his ear, and whisper sexual fantasies to him if you want to shorten the process. This is one reason you should have your head right next to his.

5) How tightly do you grip? Put three fingers in your mouth, and purse your lips around them. Now purse your lips (NOT your teeth) as tightly as you can. THAT is how tightly you should hold his shaft in your hand. If you are gripping it the right tightness, then you should feel the irregularities that lie under the skin of his penis. A mans penis is not smooth under his skin! And the sensations my hand feels as it caresses his shaft, sensing the little bumps and textures there, is a real turn on for me. Enjoy!

6) When he is beginning to stiffen throughout his body, and breathing harder, DONT speed up. Wait, make him suffer as his body begins to beg for release. When his penis begins to swell slightly, and his balls begin to pulse, put your head in his lap and tell him out-loud to cum in your mouth. Then put your lips around his cock and enjoy his gift to you. You will feel his gratitude, you will see it in his eyes, you will experience it the next day, ALL day. Men love it when you are willing

to take their cummies into your mouth and swallow them, or kiss him with it still in your mouth (ask first about that part). Personally, a mans cum is my favorite food group, full of protein and goodness!

You my have heard about the woman that liked peanut butter so well she smeared it all over her husbands cock? She liked that so well that pretty soon she didnt need the peanut butter.

Tips on Cunnilingus, Fellatio and Orgasms!

If you are wondering what I am going to share with you, then you are definitely in need of this article, especially after reading my teaser up there. I have shared many of my thoughts with you during the past few months. Mostly about females why's and woe's. I have had many men request that I give them more information on exactly what women like in the sex, and feelings department.

OK, well I will do what I do best, just simply share what my thoughts on these subjects are. Take them or leave them!

There are so many sites out there that are about dating, relationships, how to score, how to win, and yet men are still looking for answers. Why is that? Maybe it's because not every answer fits every women! That may be your first hint guys. We are all different, what works on one women will make another women slap your face with disgust. So I would think that a good thing to do is to just chat a bit with the lady and get to know the side of her that she is willing to show you. Hopefully you are smart enough to listen to her, and learn as she talks. Oh, and please save the checking out her boobs or her butt until after you have won the first battle.

I truly believe men are so quickly blinded by our physical protrusions (wink) that they immediately lose their focus at first base. Guys, the body parts are not going anywhere. Have some class and be patient. OK, enough about that very somber subject. I will leave that for another show, as they say.

Women's feelings, as most men have already experienced are nothing to joke about. Women are sensitive creatures and at the same time very strong. Those two characteristics are nothing short of explosive. The beneficial side to these hard to deal with emotions is that women are just as equally passionate and loving towards the male gender. It is our passion that fuels our desires to be wanted by men. We send off certain signals that entice and attract men. Women know exactly how to win a mans heart. Remember, we are the more sensitive feeling being, of the two genders. We also deal with hormones that turn us into monsters one minute and little tiny babies in another. Our feelings are usually on the top of our skin. That's why we get hurt so much easier than men. We are child bearers, and that instinctively causes us to be more cautious and rely on our intuitions more than facts. So guys , please forgive us for being the more feeling human. Do not hate us for it, or get frustrated with us, but love us and know that for all the pain we share, we also share twice as much pleasure. That brings me to my next thought!

Sex, that is definitely a good thought not to mention a very fun act between men and women. Women love to be touched, and felt. She wants to feel your hands on her body. It is a very important physical connection that sends messages to her most intimate senses. When a man touches a woman's body, she feels wanted, she feels lusted, she feels craved, but most of all she feels SEXY! Her self-esteem will ROAR! That my dear sweet men, is exactly the point you want her at. You want her to feel SEXY!

Women do vary with having their breasts played with. This should be done gently at first, so to not turn her off. Some women love a very passionate kiss. A passionate kiss can be an instant orgasm. Women love to feel the sensation of your breathe on thier skin. That will surely send her to a new level of sensations. Women have very sensitive backs.

A women's spine will tingle with the slightest touch of your finger tips. Kiss her shoulders, please. Kiss her belly! Kiss her thighs, that is another very sweet spot for women! Kiss her between her legs! She will be warm already, anticipating the sensation of your tongue! It is a very sweet way to taste the women that you desire! She will feel that much more open to you, knowing that you want every part of her body! Women`s bodies have so many sensations that it does take them a bit more time to get them to have an orgasm. The more sensations that you can get a women to feel, the higher she will go into her orgasm zones. Spend time tasting her, never rush her. Also please no not wear out just one spot. Women know there good spots, ask her to tell you what feels good. Be patient though, women do have a harder time talking about sex. Listen to her moans, read her body language, feel her wetness. All these are signs being sent to you. That's a plus for you also. The more orgasmic a women feels, the more adventurous she will be when it is you she wants to devour.

Remember, to tell her how SEXY she is and how sweet she tastes! Let her know how good she feels to you. Let her know that she is driving you crazy. Women also love to know that for sure. When men are quiet during sex, women feel that they are not exciting or sexy. Women need to hear that men want them and want to please them. When women feel they are wanted, that in turn makes them want to please their man. HMMM! Where do you think my thoughts are going now??

MHM!! Women also love to please their men. They know that men crave fellatio, better know to most as ,"Blow-jobs". (SMilz) Yes guys we know, we know. Women read more that you can imagine how just how to give their guy the best BJ. There are just as many books out there and sites on the internet about that as there are about how to please a woman. My hint to all the women wondering out there is...PRACTICE!!!! Body language from your man is a must to watch for. Not all men are the same. Some men are more sensitive in some areas that others. Just as women are also on different levels of sensations when it comes to oral sex. Another good tip ladies is your thoughts at the time of the Bj. Think sex. Think wet.Think suction. Think warm. Think HIM!! Love him!! But most of all suck him like you want it. The more he feels that you are just absolutely crazy for it, the more intense it is for him. Do not be afraid of what you are doing. You cannot hurt him unless you bite. That's a NO! NO!.... DO NOT BITE or SCRAPE! Don`t be afraid to ask him how it feels, or if there is anything more you can do to please him.

Communication, as in anything, is important in sex. It is after all, something that we want to enjoy with one another. Also we learn more about each other through sharing our physical desires. Ladies another very huge turn on for your man is when he sees you feel SEXY! When a man sees his woman sexy, confident and open to him, it will totally send him over the edge of lust for you. So lets get SEXY!!

When all is said and done, Cuddles is a biggie. We need to cuddle. It reassures us that everything was perfect. It's kind of like the icing on the cake. It bonds us on another level of communication. Some women and men have their best conversations when they cuddle. It is almost like a surrender of weapons.

Well these are my thoughts on this. I hope I have not offended anyone. I know this is a different subject than what you are use to reading. But I am human also, just like you. Also I wanted to show a little attitude of a different color for my readers.

Enjoy life and enjoy all of its benefits.

We only get but one shot at it.

Men and Women were made to enjoy each other.

So just do it!

Threesome Tips

First of all you should have a clear idea of what you expect from this experience and try to make a plan of actions. All that preplanning will help you to avoid the mistakes and to enjoy your threesome experience fully.

Usually the most desirable for men type of threesome is with two women. Some men include their girlfriend or wives in threesome activities, the others dont. Well, it all depends on your imagination and sexuality.

When dealing with this kind of threesome a man should understand that the comfort of his woman (if she is involved) must be his first and major objective. This kind of experience with affect your relationships for sure, therefore try to avoid anything that would be uncomfortable for her. Keep in mind that you should give your woman the most of your attention in order not to cause her being jealous. Assure your girlfriend that she is your prior concern and its a pure experiment for fun.

Never forget about safety. Use different condom for each partner and different hands for pleasuring each woman. For safety reasons it is better not to swap hands. The same safety rules are applicable if you use different sex toys during your play. Apply a separate condom for every toy when using it on each partner.

The common misconception about threesome with two women and a man is that a man is a center and gets all the attention from both women. Having these expectations you may feel a little bit ignored because your women will be also busy pleasuring each other as well. Its not you who gets the most of attention. It is more like a cycle activity, sex moves from person to person and the wisest thing here is to be as generous and giving as possible and you will get all the attention in return. Concentrate on pleasuring your women and eventually you will get the rewards.

There will be moments when you might feel completely abandoned, when two women are pleasuring each other. Instead of simply watching them, get yourself involved. You can pleasure yourself during these breaks of course, but there are much more exiting things to do. See what you can do. If one of the women is positioned comfortably to give oral sex, take the initiative. Or you can also caress their breasts, backs, inner thighs. Forget about your feelings, get sensual.

Another difficulty that you may face is the penetration. When you are penetrating one woman the other is left on her own, that is why you should make sure that both women agree on that. But even the penetration is different in threesome. Its no one on one sex; all three of you should get the attention. So, when penetration one woman you can give some attention to the other, for example talk dirty to her, caress her with your hands, kiss her, etc.

More likely that you will get overexcited from threesome experience and come more quickly than usual, but dont forget to make sure that both women are satisfied, you must make both of women climax by any means.

Also keep in mind that it is just a sexual experiment not a relationship. But if dont feel confident about trying threesome, dont try to relax by drinking for bravery, as usually it ends up in a sore morning disappointment.

Therefore all three of you must feel comfortable with the idea of having a threesome experience.

That is the only way it is going to work and give you exciting sexual experience.

The World Naked Bike Ride Experience

I had not heard of the World Naked Bike Ride (WNBR) until a couple of weeks before this year's events in June when I accidently came across the websites while doing research with Google for my article writing for SexTingles.

I have been a naturist for many years. The one thing about us British that niggles me is the ambivalent nature we have generally about sex. It means that, despite the modern day openness in the media, people are still usually very reserved about their own sex lives. This is mixed with an apparently insatiable desire to hear about other people's sex lives; particularly those of celebrities. There is a continual hypocritical outcry about the sexual behaviour of celebrities and politicians plastered across the news media and tut-tutted at by all and sundry although most of those doing the tut-tutting are 'carrying on' in much the same way.

So what has all this to do with the WNBR? Well first of all British Naturists are some of the nicest people there are, but they are also some of the most sexually confused/scared/hypocritical. Society being what it is has always been very wary of the idea and practice of naturism – because the mere state of being naked with other human beings has sexual connotations. Naturists have responded by denying any sexual aspect in their social nakedness. It is of course true that for most people sexy clothing can be even more of a turn-on than full nakedness and if you are habitually naked among other people you become used to the sight of naked bodies and peoples' genitals. However, in my opinion, if one naturist is attracted to another, their nakedness can and should be a 'turn-on'.

This sets the stage for the WNBR. Non-naturists braving public nakedness for the 'cause'; naturists many in denial about the possible sexual nature of nakedness and the non-naturist public titilated by the thought and sight of nakedness and driven by a hypocritical convention to love and condemn, at the same time, public nakedness and sexuality.

Against this background the WNBR is first and foremost a light-hearted event to present a serious protest against the dependency on fossil fuels, the dangers of overuse of cars both to the environment and to cyclists, and the benefit of cycling to people and the environment. Rides are run throughout the world over the same few days in June. The rides are billed as naked (though there is no insistence on participants being fully naked) to draw attention to the vulnerability of the human body to pollution and cars – and of course to attract the attention of the public.

As usual with these events the Brighton Group discussed arrangements with the local police who were helpful and did not see any problem with riders being naked. However, just days before the event the Assistant Chief Constable intervened and pronounced that riders would be arrested if they, in his words, "exposed their 'rude bits'". Apart from the dubious legality of this directive (perhaps the subject of another article) does this (panic?) act not show the confusion society has about morality, sexuality and nakedness! Was it his own opinion that he was imposing, was it the result of pressure from some very influential person or people, did he really believe that the general public would really be significantly offended and up in arms over the nakedness? The organisers advised partipants to use imaginative ideas to cover up – exactly what was not clear. Would bare buttocks and breasts be OK?

When the day arrived my nervousness intensified. Not because I would be (nearly) naked but because I was anxious about the public's reaction, especially as I had a panel on the bike declaring being sponsored by SexTingles and supporting both WNBR and the Outsiders Club. Would they be offended; would they laugh at us or would they be supportive? Would the other riders be uncomfortable with my sponsorship (with its sexual connections)?

When I arrived at the Level, preparations were already underway with people doing body painting promoting the WNBR messages. I was pleased to see there was an even number of men and women (also one or two children with their parents and a dog in a bike trailer!). One or two people (men) were fully naked there were a lot of naked buttocks and breasts. More and more people arrived; the press arrived and quite few people gave interviews including myself. Then suddenly the police arrived in cars and a police van ... how were they going to react?

In the event, the police were friendly. They chatted to people and slowly and quietly talked to those who were obviously intending to go on the ride fully naked, telling them they should cover up their genitals. Mine were covered with an amusing 'elephant' thong!

At last the ride got underway and around 160 riders left the park area and with the help of the police who directed at traffic lights and junctions we travelled down the Steine to the the Brighton Palace Pier and then along the seafront to Hove. The public reaction seemed mixed with amusement and bemusement. Quite a few cheered us on our way. At the Statue of Peace we waited for the stragglers to catch up. Then we turned north into the shopping areas and cycled along Western Road and past Churchill Square. It was in this area that we past the most people. Again most were supportive. A few older people ignored us or turned away and looked uncomfortable, but no-one showed any signs of being really upset.

The ride then took us east through Kemptown and then finally back down to the sea at the Brighton Naturist Beach. There people gathered to take a rest and have some lunch. A few of the riders then went back into Brighton to catch a train up to London to take part in the London ride – which actually did have fully naked riders!

There were only two instances of note. At one point the police held up traffic to let us through but at the head of the queue was a bus. The bus driver was so annoyed at being held up he moved forward and used the bus to push the policeman out of the way – he got a good talking to! One of the riders arrived at the finish in the police van; but he had not been arrested, in fact he had had a puncture and the police gave him a lift!

Since the event I have read a few responses from the public, some of whom maintain it must have been an illegal act as it "destroyed the Queen's Peace" others applauding it and yet others arguing the case for cycling and cars and the use of the roads. Hopefully the ride did get people thinking about the issues, although to my mind the problems and cures are not as simple as such a protest tends to suggest.

So, an event that I had been anxious about turned out to be great fun and all the people taking part were very friendly. I took part to help save the World and would not have missed it for the World!

The Truth About Sexual Power

Prostitution has been called "the world's oldest profession". That truth is based on a power imbalance which derives from the physical nature of human bodies. Simply put, women have an opening in their bodies that men need permission to get into and whenever permission is required for something important, the person who gets to give permission has power over the person who has to ask for permission. Furthermore, women have several other physical features that men strongly desire, while men really only have one major feature that women truly need. The result of that power imbalance is that women can almost always get some kind of sex when they want it and men cannot do the same thing. If a woman walks into a bar or club and beckons "come here" with her first finger, every man who can still stand up will jump at the opportunity. If a man were to do the same thing, the female yawn would be deafening.

In ancient Greece, a classic play was written called "The Trojan Women". It took place in the City of Troy, and at that time, all the men were warriors who were constantly leaving their wives to go off to fight in various battles in foreign lands. The Greek wives in those days did not even think about cheating on their husbands and like all women, they had powerful sexual needs but their needs could not be met because their husbands were not there to do it for them. As their sexual frustration increased to an intolerable level, they became more and more unhappy about the situation. One day the wives called a city meeting to discuss their problem and they all agreed on a very simple solution. They decided to withhold all sexual favors from their husbands until every single one of the men agreed to stop going off to war once and for all. When the husbands came home to their wives and wanted to have sex with them, they couldn't believe the situation they were confronted with. Of course they got extremely angry and even violent about it. But every single one of the wives stuck to the agreement they had made with each other and none of them surrendered to their violent husbands. The eventual result was that the husbands caved in to the will of their wives and they all agreed to stop the wars. Too bad American women are not prepared to do the same thing.

Many people believe that men have the power in this world simply because they are bigger than woman and physically stronger than women. Of course, men have always been willing to use their overwhelming physical strength to dominate and control women. But while it is generally true that men are physically stronger than women, there is an even more powerful truth behind that truth which was dramatized by "The Trojan Women". Have you ever heard the old saying, "Behind every powerful man, there is a woman"? Hitler had Eva Braun, and even Mickey Mouse had Minnie. Exceptions to that rule are male homosexuals who achieve positions of power and a very few powerful men who never marry or have long term relationships.

Ever since the beginning of recorded human history, men have found two simple solutions to their problem of intolerable sexual frustration. I don't include happily married men who are able to maintain their marriages without ever cheating, but I am including the married men who do cheat. The vast majority of divorces are directly related to infidelity, and most of it is committed by men. One solution men found before recorded history began is rape, which they do not need permission for, and male anger over the power imbalance is certainly one of the reasons behind rape. Please don't mistake me – I believe rape is an inexcusable violation of women's natural human rights. The other solution for men is prostitution and it is extremely common for men to use prostitutes so that they can live out fantasies which they cannot or will not enjoy with their wives. Women discovered that they could use the power imbalance to solve a big problem for themselves, and it's not a sexual problem. Throughout history, women were simply not allowed by men to earn money by working at a job but they could make money secretly by being prostitutes. An unspoken agreement was formed which worked for both sides and that's the reason why prostitution has flourished in all societies even though it is almost always against the law. Nowadays women are able to earn money by using their non-sexual talents and abilities, but many women still choose to do it by renting their bodies and that's self evident because of the great number of very intelligent prostitutes. I'm not saying that prostitution is an easy job, but historically it was the only money making job available to women.

Pornography is a relatively new development in human history because it really began to flourish after the development of the Kodak camera. Prior to the invention of photographs, all that existed were drawings created by horny men who were not very good artists. Many women believe that pornography is all about degradation of women by men who are exploiting them. Betty Page, the very first photographed "pin-up girl", would have disputed that theory from her own personal experience. Betty discovered that she was extremely turned on by being photographed in sexy poses. Men quickly discovered an almost universal desire to look at photographs of nude women. Almost immediately after Betty's photos were published, many other women discovered the same desire in themselves and began to fantasize about being able to do the same thing that Betty did.

Hugh Hefner was in the right place at the right time with the right concept, and he accumulated an enormous fortune by publishing the first mass magazine that featured beautiful nude women. Do you remember who the first centerfold was? It was Marilyn Monroe. Marilyn was already becoming a movie star and she certainly didn't need to put herself out to the public that way. Within a very short amount of time, other pornographic magazines sprung into existence because so many men were jealous of Hefner and were attempting to do the same thing. There was never a shortage of willing female models and it's ridiculous to believe that all of them allowed themselves to be degraded. By the late 1970's, video production exploded and pornography moved into the new medium because it is so much more expressive than photographs can possibly be. Many female pornographic superstars were created by the new medium. Just ask Annie Sprinkes, Candy Samples, or Ushi Digart why they participated in so many of the early classic porno videos. Their answers would be the same, and Annie is actually a philosopher on the subject. Annie believes that it's all about female self expression that results in freedom and independence from male domination.

One serious problem for prostitutes has traditionally been how to get paying clients without the risk of physical danger. The newest solution to that problem is the internet. The number of women who have posted pornographic photos to the internet is beyond calculation and there are a prodigious number of prostitutes who have discovered its safe marketing power. By using the internet, many prostitutes are able to earn well over $100,000 per year and they don't even have to accept a client who does not physically attract them. Talk about sexual power! There are countless personal web sites where women are collecting clients like Japanese fishermen who drag mile long nets through the ocean picking up every single fish who are caught by the net (net pun intended).

I rest my case. (in case I ever get some rest about all this)

The sexual revolution

The sexual revolution came in the 1960s with the concept of free love promoted by the hippies. During this time, the knowledge of human sexuality was redefined as the introduction of psychedelic drugs and a counter-culture that rejected traditional ways and upheld individual freedom. It was in this period of history we see nude coeds in the streets. Horny coeds were seen fucking in the streets. Different terms emerged as new activities were developed. Free love was operationalized as sex anywhere, anytime, with anyone and without guilty. Women were liberated because of the introduction of the contraceptive pill. Now they were no longer confined as mothers and wives. This too, gave them greater control over their reproductive functions. They can now engage in coed sex without worrying about the consequences.

In 1948, the release of the Kinsey report opened the minds of many Americans to the diversity of sexual behaviors not only in the United States but also around the world. It was during this time that bisexuals, gays and lesbians were first recognized. According to the report, at that time, 10% of the population was gay. This was the first time that homosexuality was put in the limelight. It was also during this time that a great number of people admitted to masturbating. Sex was at last, a topic to discuss. An advance in the issue of sex came in the 1950s when a clinical study of Human Sexual Responses discussed the topics of vaginal orgasm and pre-come.

These studies paved way for greater expression of sexuality and the experimentation on sensuality and sex as a special component to living life to the fullest. Rock and roll became the language of the revolution as it began expressing the hidden desires of adults and adolescents alike. We will remember that the children of this time were called baby boomers and teens, as well as college students were allowed to sexually experiment with people who are their age, other times, older.

In our modern world, it is noted by researchers that another sexual revolution is about to happen. This is what they all as the teen sexual revolution. In 1991, a TV show entitled Doggie Howser, M.D. featured the many issues that an 18-year old needs to face in todays society. The show, aimed at preteen and teenage kids showed this teenagers life as he relinquished his virginity. The episode which showed him having sex with his teen college girlfriend also had the highest rating for the season. It seems that even in these times, the effect of the 1960s sexual revolution is still very much felt. Evidently, baby boomers can still be found today, and they take their forms as teenagers.

The Sexual Body Feelings and Erogenous Zones of Men

There is a widespread misunderstanding by many women, and surprisingly also by many men that boys and men only have sexual feelings in their penis, or even only in their penis head. The reason why many men also carry this misconception is probably that boys often are educated to suppress corporeal sensations and to be hard.

Many erogenous zones in men and boys are best activated when the body is relaxed, and the zones are stimulated in a gentle manner. Gentle stimulation of these zones in a relaxed state can give feelings of pleasure as strong as those in the penis, and can even result in some types of strong orgasmic reactions. Here is a survey of various erotic zones in the male body, and how to stimulate the sensations in these zones. You can stimulate yourself at these zones when masturbating, or the your female or gay partner can do the stimulation work.

THE SCROTUM AND THE TESTICLES

The scrotal skin and the content of the scrotum, including the testicles, are sensitive to erotic stimulation. When stimulating these genital parts, take first hold of the scrotum with your whole hand, warming it inside your hand, and massaging it gently by gripping movements. Warming and handling the scrotum gives feelings in the whole genital region. Stimulation of the scrotum also increases the blood circulation and engorgement of all the genital organs around the scrotum. The testicles are best stimulated by gentle rolling movements with your fingers. Also tickle the scrotal skin with your finger tips. A part of the penis is actually hidden partly inside and partly behind the scrotal sack, by palpating with your finger tips between the testicles or at the side under the scrotum; you can massage this part of the penis. A sharp massage with your finger tips gives the most intense sensations to this hidden root of the penis.

THE BREAST NIPPLES AND THEIR SURROUNDINGS

The nipples of a man are important erogenous zones, and a man has tits just as a woman, although the tits of a man are smaller and flatter that those of a woman. Actually a man has all the structures that a woman has in his breasts, but they are not developed to have a milk producing capacity. This means that a mans breasts have the same erotic capacity as the tits of woman. A man's nipples also have an erective capacity. They rise and get hard upon stimulation. When stimulating a mans breasts, take hold of the breast with your whole hand, warming it inside your hand, and massaging it gently by gripping movements. To stimulate the nipples, massage gently around the nipples with a finger tip. Also squeeze the nipples with your fingers, varying the intensity from the very gentle nip to some harder pressure.

THE REGION BETWEEN THE PENIS AND THE ANUS

The visible penis is actually a part of a larger body beginning at the prostate region just in front of the anus, and reaches to the tip of the penis. The urethra also goes through this structure. The parts between your legs will engorge when you are sexually exited just as the penis, and when it engorges, the region bulges out between the legs. Upon mechanical stimulation, this area gives intense pleasurable feelings. You can stimulate this area by squeezing it between your fingers, pressing down against the urethra or massaging up and down along the urethra. You should change between gentle and a little harder handling, as these two manners give rise to different types of feelings.

THE NAVEL AND THE BLADDER REGION

The navel is an erotic point, and so are the structures in the middle of the belly between the navel and the penis. This structure contains a groove between the belly muscles. The structures in this groove are very sensuous, the so called linea alba. The naval can be stimulated by sticking a finger into it, and by tickling with your finger deep down in the navel. Also here you should alternate between light, gentle, slow tickling, and harder sharper tickling. This stimulation give sensations that radiate out form the navel to the surroundings, and spreads downwards to the tip of your penis, giving a very funny feeling in your penis. The groove between the navel and the penis, you can stimulate by massaging up and down with the tip of your fingers.

THE BUTTOCKS AND ANAL SURROUNDINGS

The inner sides of the buttocks in the natal cleft give rise to deep erotic feelings with a very special intimate valor. Move your fingers up and down between the buttocks from the spine to the opposite end between the legs, and gently massage the inner side of each buttock with your finger tips. You can also concentrate your attention to the region deep inside the cleft very near the anus and tickle these most intimate points with your finger tips. Further you can stretch each buttock to the side so that the butt cleft opens, and the rectal opening is also stretched. The result of these manipulations is erotic sensations that radiate to the whole pelvic area, flow deep inside you and rise upwards along your spine.

THE ANUS AND THE OUTER RECTUM

The anal region is in many ways the real central of feelings in a man or boy. By stimulating this area in the proper ways, you can create a process that spread waves of intense feelings of joy, pleasure and ecstasy up through the whole body, partly forward to the genitals and belly region, and partly along the spine up to the neck. You best stimulate the rectal opening by very gentle circulatory movements with your finger tips. Alternate between these circulatory movements and the stimulation of the insides of the buttocks. You can also stick a smeared finger into the anal opening and stimulate by gentle movements in and out. By sticking your finger further inside, you can gently massage the inside walls of the anus. By adding some pressure, your stimulation reaches deep into the tissue around the rectum. All these stimulation give rise to profound feelings radiating to the whole body.

THE DEEP PART OF THE RECTUM

The perhaps most intimate and sensitive zone of a man, is the deep part of the rectum. This zone can be reached by gay intercourse or with a dildo or some other long object. When inserting something in the anus to stimulate this zone, it is necessary to be very cautious so that the intestinal walls are not hurt. However, this zone is so sensitive that even the gentlest stimulation gives an immense depth of feelings, both of physical and psychological kind. You can stimulate this zone by gently and gradually by inserting a thin smeared dildo, and when fully inserted, very gently move it a little in and out, a little around, or press gently to different sides with the dildo. The more you relax, and the longer you do this stimulation, the deeper and more intense will the feelings grow.

THE PROSTATE:

The prostate lies just in front of the anus and the urethra goes through it. This gland produces much of the viscous fluid in the semen. You can stimulate it from the outside by pressing somewhat firmly with your fingers inward just in front of the anus. There is a deepening in this area, just like a little vagina. Press your finger into this groove and a little forward. You can also stimulate the prostate by inserting your finger into the anus and massage the prostate through the front wall of the anus. The massage releases prostate fluid. Feeling the fluid coming through your urethra and dripping out through you pee-hole, add to the physical excitement. Also the prostate have its own sexual feelings, and prostate massage combined with anal stimulation can induce a form of orgasm that has a much deeper psychological and ecstatic impact than ordinary penile orgasm.

The Rise of Adult Movies on Demand

Pornographic films first gained attention back in the early 1900s which is what has paved the way for the rising popularity of adult movies on demand. Since pornographic films are pictures with the sole purpose of promoting sexual arousal in the viewer, it makes sense why adult movies on demand have become a mainstay in homes across the world.

Adult movies are just about as old as the medium itself. The very first pornographic motion picture that can be dated for sure is A LEcu d Or ou la bonne auberge and was made in France in 1908. The story is about a tired, weary soldier who ends up having a tryst with a young girl who works at an inn. This was about a hundred years ago and the impact of it continues to be felt today. Adult films were very popular during the era of silent movies in the 1920s and were typically shown in brothels.

There are many different classifications that fall under the umbrella of pornographic films. There are adult films, stag films, softcore porn and hardcore. Adult and stag films are older ways of referring to pornography and are not used as much anymore. Softcore typically refers to a type of film that does not show any sort of penetration or extreme fetish acts. Hardcore pornography is just the opposite and depicts sexual activities on any level.

While adult films have become much more accepted in society, there is still and probably always will be, a negative feeling attached to it. As long as there are conservative minds inhabiting the world, this will always be the case. Many people view pornography as perverted and dirty. This alone has made those who do watch it feel ashamed and embarrassed, always having to be discreet and secretive. This makes it very difficult to go out to a store and purchase films without feeling nervous that someone may see you and silently judge you. This has made for a very welcomed introduction of adult movies on demand. This allows people to purchase pornographic films in the comfort of their own home. Adult movies on demand give people the privacy they want and make watching adult films an enjoyable experience once again. The films can be bought over the internet or even through an On Demand service available through a local cable provider. Gone are the days filled with shame and embarrassment, say hello to the new age of adult movies on demand.

The quest for liberation and rights recognition

Have you ever heard of the term LGBT or GLBT to some? Well, this is actually a collective term used to refer to lesbians, gays, bisexuals and transsexuals. When you hear the term gay culture, it usually refers to them.

The sexual revolution was said to have occurred in the 1960s and up until then, the LGBT community were referred to as the third gender or the third sex. Nowadays, people call members of this community as homosexuals or homos which in itself is a derogatory term.

In the past, bisexuals and transsexuals were not considered as a part of this community as they were believed to be nothing as men or women who were afraid to come out and admit their identities. This view started right after the Stonewall riots in the late 1970s to early 1980s. It was only in the 1990s that bisexuals and transsexuals were included in what we now call as the gay community.

Since then, the cry for liberation and the acceptance of the rights of the LGBT has been a constant debate among scholars, the church and lay people. Despite the widespread integration of LGBT communities to mainstream culture, it is undeniable that some people are apprehensive with the thought of having a neighbor who is lesbian or gay.

In the United Kingdom, a TV series entitled Queer as Folk rocked the whole world as it features the many problems encountered by gay people in their daily lives. It also shows the enticing night life that they experience and the fanfare of celebrations hosted by anyone belonging to the community. We also see the many stereotypes associated with gay people in general the myths and the truths the proliferation of drugs, sex and alcohol.

This is perhaps the reason why people look at gay individuals as immoral and undeserving of praise. If normal people can do things such as watch pornographic material and nobody has any qualms, a gay person caught watching gay sample video is regarded as lowly. This is something I do not understand. Gay people are individuals who have their own rights and are hoping for their own voice. If straight people can appear in adult films, why cant gays appear in gay web cam sites? Sure we are in a sexual revolution, but this revolution is characterized more by the liberation of women than by those belonging to the subculture of the gay community.

A lot of times society treats people unfairly. A lot of the members of LGBT do something good for their community but no one notices. Maybe we think that it was their duty to pay off their mistakes. But that is blatantly cruel and unjust.

The Porno Goddess Savannah Stern

Well known in the fetish genre of the adult entertainment world, Savannah Stern stars in several films from foot fetish features to gangbangs and even violently themed porno flicks that depict women fighting with one another. Within the adult entertainment industry and world of pornography, producers and actors strive to offer every sort of genre or theme of porn, which is smart in a niche market. Men and women alike enjoy a varieties of porno films or adult entertainment films and even videos on demand, websites and magazines which depict not only hardcore sex scenes but also hardcore sex scenes with a fetish theme.

Savannah Stern is one such adult film entertainer and actress who is featured in catfight themed flicks. Catfight themed flicks make up a unique genre of adult entertainment material available across several mediums including magazine, online video, and video on demand. Men and women who are excited by this genre of porn like to see women battling it out and then kissing and making up, perhaps in a hot lesbian sex scene with dildos, anal action, strap on toys and of course more tongue and oral action than most people could handle in real life. Some such films get wild with their scenarios such as catfights where multiple women are wrestling in the mud. Dirty in so many ways, muddy women, naked and dirty, glistening in earthly juices then go on to angry sex scenes where more angry talk and dirty talk transpires.

Savannah Stern also stars in foot fetish films due to the cuteness of her feet. Some men and women particularly like to smell, lick and rub feet all over their bodies as a form of foreplay, during masturbation, or even while actual penetration is taking place. This is in fact considered hardcore porn action if the penetration can be seen in the films content. Perhaps the reason men and women develop foot fetishes is because, like most other erogenous parts of the body, although feet are not considered so erogenous, they are covered up and hidden most of the time, so the excitement of seeing something one normally would not can have the ability to sexually arouse, stimulate and eventually make foot enthusiasts cum hard.

Group sex scenes, also known as gang bangs or orgies, is also a popular adult entertainment genre favorite among those who fantasize about sexual relations with more than one person at a time. Savannah Stern the sexy adult film star is either the star or featured actress in several such mentioned genres of porno.

The Natural Roots of Sexuality

Recent studies in animal sexuality serve to dispel two common myths: that sex is exclusively about reproduction and that homosexuality is an unnatural sexual preference. It now appears that sex is also about recreation as it frequently occurs out of the mating season. And same-sex copulation and bonding are common in hundreds of species, from bonobo apes to gulls.

Moreover, homosexual couples in the Animal Kingdom are prone to behaviors commonly – and erroneously – attributed only to heterosexuals. The New York Times reported in its February 7, 2004 issue about a couple of gay penguins who are desperately and recurrently seeking to incubate eggs together.

In the same article ("Love that Dare not Squeak its Name"), Bruce Bagemihl, author of the groundbreaking "Biological Exuberance: Animal Homosexuality and Natural Diversity", defines homosexuality as "any of these behaviors between members of the same sex: long-term bonding, sexual contact, courtship displays or the rearing of young."

Still, that a certain behavior occurs in nature (is "natural") does not render it moral. Infanticide, patricide, suicide, gender bias, and substance abuse – are all to be found in various animal species. It is futile to argue for homosexuality or against it based on zoological observations. Ethics is about surpassing nature – not about emulating it.

The more perplexing question remains: what are the evolutionary and biological advantages of recreational sex and homosexuality? Surely, both entail the waste of scarce resources.

Convoluted explanations, such as the one proffered by Marlene Zuk (homosexuals contribute to the gene pool by nurturing and raising young relatives) defy common sense, experience, and the calculus of evolution. There are no field studies that show conclusively or even indicate that homosexuals tend to raise and nurture their younger relatives more that straights do.

Moreover, the arithmetic of genetics would rule out such a stratagem. If the aim of life is to pass on one's genes from one generation to the next, the homosexual would have been far better off raising his own children (who carry forward half his DNA) – rather than his nephew or niece (with whom he shares merely one quarter of his genetic material.)

What is more, though genetically-predisposed, homosexuality may be partly acquired, the outcome of environment and nurture, rather than nature.

An oft-overlooked fact is that recreational sex and homosexuality have one thing in common: they do not lead to reproduction. Homosexuality may, therefore, be a form of pleasurable sexual play. It may also enhance same-sex bonding and train the young to form cohesive, purposeful groups (the army and the boarding school come to mind).

Furthermore, homosexuality amounts to the culling of 10-15% of the gene pool in each generation. The genetic material of the homosexual is not propagated and is effectively excluded from the big roulette of life. Growers – of anything from cereals to cattle – similarly use random culling to improve their stock. As mathematical models show, such repeated mass removal of DNA from the common brew seems to optimize the species and increase its resilience and efficiency.

It is ironic to realize that homosexuality and other forms of non-reproductive, pleasure-seeking sex may be key evolutionary mechanisms and integral drivers of population dynamics. Reproduction is but one goal among many, equally important, end results. Heterosexuality is but one strategy among a few optimal solutions. Studying biology may yet lead to greater tolerance for the vast repertory of human sexual foibles, preferences, and predilections. Back to nature, in this case, may be forward to civilization.

The Importance of Female Clitoral Orgasm

By far the most common way for a woman to regularly reach orgasm is through direct or indirect clitoral stimulation. Before we just into that subject, I think it may help to share with you some information about the clitoris.

The clitoris is located just by the vaginal entrance and behind the labia minora. In most women, it is a small nub of flesh which contains a high concentration of nerve endings which make it highly sensitive. It is often covered by a clitoral hood. Many people don't realize that only a small portion of the clitoris is actually visible. The remainder of the organ is surrounded by the rest of the reproductive system and extends all the way to the bottom of the pubic bone.

Two things are particularly interesting about the clitoris. First, all female mammals have a clitoris. This is interesting because the sole purpose, at least according to biologists, of the clitoris is sexual pleasure. That would seem to mean that humans aren't the only ones who enjoy the way sex feels.

Second, the clitoris is made from the same material as the penis. In fact, in men the clitoris becomes a full-fledged penis after the embryo is exposed to testosterone in the womb. Just like the penis, the clitoris fills with blood and becomes erect during sexual arousal. The clitoral hood is essentially the same as the foreskin of a penis.

Second, the clitoris is made from the same material as the penis. In fact, in men the clitoris becomes a full-fledged penis after the embryo is exposed to testosterone in the womb. Just like the penis, the clitoris fills with blood and becomes erect during sexual arousal. The clitoral hood is essentially the same as the foreskin of a penis.

What many people don't realize about the clitoris is that the penis alone usually cannot stimulate it. Because of its position in the woman's body, the ability of the penis to provide rhythmic stimulation to the clitoris is extremely difficult. That means traditional intercourse usually needs to be coupled with clitoral stimulation.

What many people don't realize about the clitoris is that the penis alone usually cannot stimulate it. Because of its position in the woman's body, the ability of the penis to provide rhythmic stimulation to the clitoris is extremely difficult. That means traditional intercourse usually needs to be coupled with clitoral stimulation.

The question is how does one engage in clitoral stimulation. Some male partners take the approach that the women should be responsible for the stimulation themselves, which has always seemed a bit unfair to me since the woman is providing him with the stimulation he needs to reach orgasm. However, this is one way to deal with it.

Other couples I've met with have resorted to an alternative approach. One person reaches orgasm at a time. Depending on how each person best reaches orgasm, this may be a possibility but it's usually not the most satisfactory approach.

Another method is by, what I like to call multi-tasking. Multi-tasking basically means the man does more than one thing at the same time. For example, he may be penetrating the vagina while also stimulating the clitoris in one way or another (we'll discuss those ways a little later). If the couple wants to achieve orgasm at or near the same time, this is clearly the best option.

The best thing about clitoral orgasms is that they can be achieved in many different ways. Because the entire area is highly sensitive, experimenting with these types of orgasms can also add some interest and spice to sexual relationships which may have become less enthusiastic over time.

And the key is experimenting because different women prefer different types of clitoral stimulation. While some prefer direct stimulation, others find it uncomfortable and prefer to have the area around the clitoris stimulated instead. Women who have masturbated will generally have a much better idea of what type of stimulation they prefer than women who have not.

As I mentioned, the clitoris feels up with blood and becomes erect like a penis. This means its usually easier to spot when a woman is aroused. Because the clitoris does not need to be erect for sexual intercourse to occur, clitoral orgasms will only happen if the woman is aroused properly. That means some type of foreplay is generally a requirement. When the clitoris is stimulated repeatedly, it becomes more engorged with blood and this further heightens its sensitivity. With another stimulation a point is reached when all of the tension in the area must be released and this point is considered the orgasm.

The History Of Pay Per View Demand

Pay per view is a system where a television viewer can purchase events that are telecast on TV and pay for it to privately air in their homes. When you purchase an event like this it is shown to everyone who orders it at the same exact time, but there is also an option known as pay per view demand. With pay per view demand, you can start the program or event you bought at any time you want. This is a nice feature because it allows you to tailor it to fit into your schedule instead of the other way around. Pay per view can be ordered using an on screen guide, an automated telephone system or with a live customer service representative. It is always nice to have the option to speak with a customer service representative because you can have any of your questions or concerns addressed right away. Although pay per view is offered through your local cable provider, it is actually considered a separate industry.

Pay per view gained its mainstream popularity mostly from sporting events. For the first time, it allowed fans to watch events that were broadcast all over the world without actually having to be there in person. The first major pay per view event took place on September 16, 1981 when Sugar Ray Leonard fought Thomas Hearns for the Welterweight Championship. A company in Nashville, Tennessee called Viacom Cablevision was the first one to offer this event and they sold more than 50% of their customers for the fight. This set quite a precedent for pay per view events in the future. They actually got Sugar Ray Leonard to visit Nashville to promote the fight which made the event such a huge success.

The term pay per view did not become widely used until the 1990s when companies like IN Demand, Showtime and HBO began using the system to broadcast their programs and movies. While boxing has always been one of the biggest things purchased through pay per view, concerts and show movies also became very popular. This is when the idea of offering pay per view demand came about because they saw an opportunity to capitalize on the popularity of pay per view. The only problem with the current pay per view system was that not everyone was available to view something at the same time. Pay per view demand gave viewers the ability to decide when they would watch a purchased event, which ultimately made subscribers much more satisfied.

The French Kiss

A kiss is a unique way of expressing emotions between couples since it is intimate, subtle, and sensual all at the same time. A good kiss lets the couple lose themselves in the heat of the moment, each reacting and reciprocating every nuance of the kiss for a really exciting experience. Different people react to different kinds of kisses, so there is no real foolproof way of giving a topnotch kiss. As long as both of the couples enjoy the experience, then that pleasure is a great kiss in itself. Kissing is greatly enhanced with the act of sexual intercourse, but before couples make contact, it is advised that they employ the use of condoms for protection. Lubricated latex condoms greatly enhance the experience while keeping the individual safe from possible transmission of diseases. Durex condoms come in different designs, flavors and scents which add further excitement to the experience.

The French kiss is a sensual open mouth kiss which involves a lot of tongue to tongue contact. There are plenty of techniques in making a French kiss especially pleasurable and exciting. Lightly caressing the lips with the tongue is a good way to start, then continuing this motion with increasing aggressiveness, as both partners react to the urgency, should take

advantage of the heat of the moment. When the tongues eventually come in contact, doing a swirling motion greatly enhances the pleasure of the kiss. The tongue could try to chase each other while occasionally coming in contact. Gentle sucking with the lips and small nibbles on the tongue in addition to tongue contact are also great ways to progress in a French kiss. Playing along and experimenting with the kiss are a pleasurable experience all by itself, and the couple are encouraged not to restrict themselves too much to rules as this self-defeats the purpose of the act. The couple should feel free to discover which technique, timing, and movements give them the most pleasure out of the experience. It is important that proper hygiene is observed for a thoroughly satisfying kiss, since bad breath is a big turn off for any one.

The Evolution From Video Cassettes To Adult Movies On Demand

The Evolution From Video Cassettes To Adult Movies On Demand

Pornographic films have an interesting history, one where attitudes have changed since the 1960s, during which time some of the first sexually explicit films were making their debut. Today, adult movies on demand are a popular commodity, and are also referred to as simply vod or even pay per view porn. What was taboo and even looked down upon may seem mild in comparison to what some adult movies on demand depict on the internet now, from interracial guy on guy sex scenes to group sex parties, orgies and fetish films where men hungrily kiss and lick and munch on womens feet, vod and pay per view porn offers horny customers a great selection of films to choose from.

It was not until 1969 that Denmark became the first country to legalize hardcore porno films. After that opinions about sexuality began to change. Leading to the rise of triple x rated porno films in United States theatres during the 1970s, people could go to a theatre in the united states, pay a cheap rate and watch a sexually explicit film. Of course this is where the joke about pop corn boxes came from. A laughable but true trick by certain horny men, in theatres some would hollow out their pop corn boxes, prop the box over their hard cocks and beat off however they pleased within the privacy of the pop corn boxes buttery, salty walls. If you remember correct, it was this pop corn box scandal that Pee Wee Herman was busted for some years later.

Adult video on demand allows horny men and women to enjoy a porno theatre experience within the comfort and privacy of their own homes. Although the theatre experience added to the thrill, masturbation in public is a punishable crime and what could be more embarrassing that getting caught in a horny, exposed, desperate state, pop corn box and dick in hand. Pay per view porn costs far less than the legal fees and blows to ones ego after being thrown in the slammer for beating ones meat in a buttery popcorn box.

Adult vod has a selection you can brose and pay for upon your tastes in hot sex scenes, and there are streaming abilities, so this is similar to a traditional movie theatre experience, in fact some kinky individuals have thrown group sex viewing parties, where adult movies on demand are projected on a big screen or even 15 foot wall. This brings quite the life to an adult pay per view porn experience.

The Bonus to Confidence Given by Penis Enlargement is Priceless

The Bonus to Confidence Given by Penis Enlargement is Priceless

Penis size is an obsession shared across generations and cultures and this obsession will not go away any time soon. From the psychological point of view, the bonus to confidence given by penis enlargement is priceless. Penis enlargement is at the pinnacle age for true aesthetic, permanent, thicker, longer wider producing penis enlargement methods. It takes time and patience to make something good in your life and penis enlargement is not an exception.

Natural penis enlargement is based on the idea that the cavernosa and spongiosum, the two pieces of spongy tissue in the penis, can be expanded to hold more blood. We understand that it can feel like you're shopping in a minefield, even once you're sure that sure that Penis Enlargement is the right choice for you. Natural Penis Enlargement is not something you can buy, it's something you need to work at. Gradual penis enlargement is the key to effective, permanent results. Penis Girth is more important than penis length because all you need is to enjoy sex whether you have small penis or big penis so if you have good girth or width then you can make your women feel and help her to release orgasms easily and both couple can enjoy their sex life.

Herbal penis enlargement is safe, affordable and guaranteed. Penis pills can help increase the blood flow to the penis tissues thus causing the penis looks bigger and harder when erected. Penis enlargement products are exceptionally safe and you can easily buy and use them from the comfort of your home. Penis enlargement has a lot of unique benefits. Your penis could be up to 2 inches bigger when using proper exercising techniques.

The fact is that penis enlargement is possible and you can increase your penis length and girth. The only other clinically proven penis enlargement

methods are medical stretching devices, such as the SizeGenetics unit. Why be content with an average penis size when perfectly natural penis enlargement is a few clicks away. The main reason why PenisHealth has been so successful was the inclusion of instructional "workout style" videos which help clients perform the needed exercises.

The Amazing Range Of Sex Toys

There are an amazing variety of sex toys available. Sex toys vary from purely male or purely female sex toys to toys that can be used by both sexes. There are also some sex toys that can also be classified as sex aids or marital aids.

The Purpose Of Sex Toys

Some sex toys aid the man's erection, stimulate the female genitals to become more sensitive or provide a different feel to 'normal' sex. Other sex toys provide an 'environment' for variations in sex, for example so called orgy bed sheets. Sometimes they are used to help a person who has difficulty with unaided sex to achieve sexual satisfaction. However most sex toys provide a new way to directly stimulate the male or female genitals to achieve sexual satisfaction.

Using sex toys can provide new experiences and variation in the sexual experience. It can also provide a fantasy element for enhancing or revitalising a relationship.

The usual expectation is that a sex toy provides direct stimulation of the genitals in foreplay and/or during sexual intercourse or as a means to obtain orgasm through only the stimulation provided by the sex toy.

Types of Sex Toys

Vibrating Sex Toys

Probably the most well known sex toys are 'vibrators' which, as the name suggests, provide stimulation of the genitals using vibration. They are mainly used to stimulate the clitoris, but may also be used to stimulate any other part of the female body or that of a man's.

The simplest of these are pencil or wand shaped (though normally thicker than a pencil). A good example is the Ceramitex vibrator. They often have an internal battery (or two) which powers a small electric motor. Sometimes the battery pack and controller are external and connected to the vibrator by a wire. This motor is fitted with a small, out of balance, weight attached to the shaft. As this weight rotates it throws the motor and vibrator into a small circular movement which causes the vibration you feel.

With a vibrator that has a controller, as the power is increased the speed of the motor increases and with it both the rate and strength of vibration. Both the strength and rate of vibration effects how stimulating you find the sex toy. The best effect may not be as strong and as fast as possible. The optimum settings may well change as your degree of excitement builds. To get the best results it is worth buying a vibrator which is controllable.

Different vibrators will have different characteristics and you may well find you prefer one combination much more than another and your preference may even vary depending on which part of your body you are stimulating.

More recently electronic vibrator controllers have appeared which provide not only the static control of power/speed but also allow you to select patterns of power pulses and surges. These can be very effective.

There are also other vibrating sex toys such as butterfly stimulators and vibrating penis rings.

Other Powered Sex Toys

There are some sex toys that use other ways to provide mechanical stimulation. These usually depend on a motor that makes the sex toy continually change its shape which provides a sort of rotational movement or makes it move back and forth. The back and forth movements are sometimes powered by an air pump rather than a motor. The movements have been used to create, for example, mechanical licking tongues, vibrators that 'penetrate' the vagina and mouth simulators to give a man a 'blow job'.

On a bigger scale and much more expensive, there are 'sex machines' that incorporate thrusting and vibrating dildos.

Combination Sex Toys

So far we have covered vibrating, moving and thrusting sex toys. As you may have guessed these are all offered in a bewildering array of combinations.

A common combination in many 'Rabbit Style' vibrators is clitoral stimulation using vibrations and vaginal stimulation using movement and sometimes a thrusting motion as well. An excellent example of these is the Hitech Crystal Fantasy vibrator.

Many sex toys add varying textures to their surfaces; a dildo or vibrator may have ridges or soft spikes or a rippled shape.

Sensation Change Sex Toys

Some sex toys rather than provide vibrating or moving stimulation, change the feel of sex.

For instance there are a variety of sleeves to put over the penis to provide different sensations for both partners while engaged in penetrative sex.

There are rings that squeeze the base of the penis and/or tighten the scrotum that assist the man's erection and also changes his sensations. There are penis extenders and thickeners which may give a man's partner greater sensations during penetration.

There are a wide variety of lubricants that can significantly change the feel of sex.

There are PVC and Polyurethane bed sheets that are water and oil proof that can be used for slippery or messy sex.

Why Use A Sex Toy?

A good question is: why do people use a sex toy? Surely fingers, tongues, penises, clitorises and vaginas etc all provide great sexual stimulation and enjoyment.

Well, apart from therapeutic uses (eg erection assistance), sex toys can drive the imagination (being taken by a machine), provide variety (new ways to do old things), vary the stimulating effects in otherwise normal sex (penis sleeves) and some can provide experiences not possible with 'normal body parts' (particularly vibrating sex toys and electro-stimulation).

Where To Start

If you have not tried a sex toy before and don't yet have an idea of what you might like, try one of the simpler vibrators first. Most probably you will enjoy the experience and then start to wonder what other delights can be found with more sophisticated vibrators and other sex toys ...

If you then find you do enjoy sex toys try out a few others and find what suits you. Above all, have fun trying them out!

The adventure of a Writer

I can say that I am a good writer. I adventure and writing about new topics. I can say Ive done pretty well considering I could write about technology, medicine and health when in fact I never studied any of these. But I found a topic, which left me speechless, or should I say wordless?

When I was asked to write about adult topics I thought we were only talking about Viagra, penis enlargement or vaginal cosmetic surgery. Topics, which, needless to say, I had no trouble writing about before. But here I am struggling to find out the definition of demand live sex and what an amateur exhibitionist does. What are fetish films and how is it different from Hollywood movies? Sure I know the difference between Hollywood and Bollywood but fetish movies are something new to me. Armed with my laptop and a liter of orange juice, I went to a public Internet shop to find the answer.

More commonly known as porn, the spread of fetish videos on the Internet has caused government bodies to introduce and implement laws limiting its reach. A lot of people are involved in public discussions and debates for and against pornography. But are these really doing any good? When censorship laws were implemented, did it really prevent the proliferation of fetish video on demand? I feel that these laws didnt really help; they only created enough noise for people to be more curious. I am not saying that porn is bad; its just that I cant see the reason for censorship laws or any evidence that pornography does any harm. Well, of course when you talk about children, pedophilia is a different world altogether.

But lets talk about pornography and why people are hooked with it. Sure someone would say: people who appear in porn films are desperate for the money, are probably drug users, criminals or prostitutes. But are these assumptions true? Someone claims: I never watched BDSM video and then proceeds to talk down on people who did. For one, how did you know about BDSM? For another, what authority do you have to judge people who happen to like watching other people doing this most basic of all necessities?

In a study conducted by Kath Albury and Catharine Lumby from the University of Sydney entitled Understanding Pornography in Australia, it was found that people like pornography because most videos reiterate that natural beauty is still most attractive for men and women alike. Also, when interviewed, people appearing in movies say that they do it because they enjoy their work. Some do it for the money, not because they are desperate but because the work is basically high-paying and safe too.

Status of Women in the Bible

How the Status of Women Changed in the Bible

Why is it that the Bible seems so unfriendly to women? After all it would appear that most of the members and committee volunteers in a congregation are female. Yet holding office, being ordained, serving in any real capacity is pretty much forbidden. Some congregations even hold up the marital status of a woman (i.e., divorced or not) as to whether or not a woman can truly advance within the denominations hierarchy.

Other than male dominance, prejudiced tradition, and/or a misunderstanding of the scriptures, why is that? The short answer is: male dominance, prejudiced tradition, and a misuse of the Bible. This short article cannot discuss male dominance or prejudiced tradition. Well focus on the misuse of the scriptures.

To read and digest the Bible we must understand several things: the mind and situation of the writer; the mind and situation of the audience; and the message the writer was trying to communicate. Having understood that, we can begin to strip away the external trappings of the writer (e.g., those elements of the Old Testament texts that clearly belong in the late Bronze Age or of the New Testament texts that clearly belong to the culture of the early first century) and concentrate on the true underlying message.

In short, just like us, the writers of biblical scripture were people of their times and their cultures. It shows.

In the Old Testament the whole concept of eternal life important in any religious system was understood as the growth and survival of ones clan or progeny. Similar to the early cultures of our Native Americans, it was the tribe or clan that was the integral unit of society not the individual. Preservation of the tribe was paramount. This was most certainly the case in the Bronze and Iron Ages of the nomadic tribes/clans of the Fertile Crescent in the mid-East known as the cradle of western civilization.

Cultural norms followed and supported that critical concept. Since men were the fighters and could impregnate more than one woman at a time, men were more expendable. For a man to have multiple wives was a sanctioned practice provided he could financially take care of them. The use of a dowry in exchange for a daughter was an integral foundation of the nomadic economy. Underlying all of this was the preeminent notion of preserving the tribe or clan.

This religious/social/economic concept worked. It was successful for a long time over 3,000 years (from 3,500 BCE to the rise of city-states under Alexander the Greats rule about 350 BCE, when urban dwelling began the slow process of breaking this down). It was not unique to the Old Testament Israelites. It was true throughout the Mesopotamian Region: Sumerians, Akkadians, Philistines, Amorites, Hittites, Babylonians, Assyrians, etc.

This patriarchal social structure is evident throughout the Old Testament and was, by our standards, very demeaning for women. Women were not much better than chattel property. Abraham had his wife Sarahs handmaiden, Hagar, after Sarah could not get pregnant. Once Sarah did get pregnant, Abraham banished Hagar and their son, Ishmael. Legend has it that mother and son are buried in Mecca and Ishmael is generally considered to be the patriarchal father of Islam. (cf. Genesis 21:8-21)

During the time of the New Testament, the role of women was denigrated during the first 100 years after the crucifixion of Jesus. We can only speculate about how and why that happened. The earliest writer in the New Testament was the Apostle Paul, who wrote between 45-55 CE. We have eight of his original letters: Galatians; I-II Thessalonians; I-II Corinthians; Philemon, Philippians; and Romans. In these letters Paul routinely praises local female parishioners in his epistles. For example, in Romans 16:1-15, he praises Phoebe, who holds office in the congregation of Cenchreae, as well as quite a few other women.

However, when he begins discussing specific congregational issues, he lets the cultural values of his Jewish upbringing show through (I Cor. 11:2-16). Yes, Paul admonishes his congregations to have womens head covered or to remain subservient to men. Yet, even so, he concludes by saying, If push comes to shove, however, we have none of these customs in a Christian congregation (I Cor 11:16). Why the confusion? I can only speculate that in the early beginnings, when congregations were meeting informally in homes, the role of the women in making that happen and in spreading the word was much more significant and critical for success. Although Paul was aware of his Jewish customs and could recommend them, it was really no big deal to him.

As these congregations grew and became more organized, the male-dominated culture took sway and women began getting pushed out. Compare Pauls letter to the Galatians (his earliest, c. 45) or his epistle to the Romans (his latest, c. 55/60) with passages like I Timothy 2:8-15, written (c.110/120) in Pauls name but decades after his death. You can see the difference. The denigration of women is even more pronounced.

However, we have to keep in mind that all of Paul s letters were written in his firm belief that the end of the world and the permanent coming of the kingdom of heaven was literally just around the corner. What I mean, my friends, is this. The time we live in will not last long. While it lasts, married men should be as if they had no wives; mourners should be as if they had nothing to grieve them, the joyful as if they did not rejoice; buyers must not count on keeping what they buy, nor those who use the worlds wealth on using it to the full. For the whole frame of this world is passing away. I Cor. 7: 29-31. Understanding this puts the onus on us to interpret all the cultural trappings of Pauls writings within the context of being intended by him as very short-term advice.

By the time of the beginning of the second century, there was a formal church organization in place. The organization consisted of various offices: Bishops (episcopoi) or overseers; elders (presbyteroi) or leaders; and deacons (diaconoi) or trusted servers of the Lord. Together these offices formed the backbone and structure of the embryonic Christian church. They were generally all male. The secondary role of women became more and more pronounced as time went by. Culturally, we can understand this. We can understand this when its reflected in scripture because we know that biblical writers reflected their times. But to ascribe this as Gods will is to misread the scripture by refusing to winnow away the cultural bias of the writers times.

We continue to maintain a second-class role for women in many of our congregations today. We refuse ordination for them as ministers or the priesthood. We maintain the subservient role they are to fill in the household. We do this by erroneously holding onto literal interpretations of the scripture when it suits us.

What can we conclude from this? Those today proclaiming the lower role for women in the church structure and citing biblical references to buttress their position are doing so more as an act of their machismo than as an exposition of biblical knowledge. Paul felt fully free to restate the accepted narrative of Israels history as he wrestled with deriving an answer to the question: Who was Jesus and why did he die? If Paul felt confident enough to reconstruct his scriptural heritage, we should have the courage to do the same. For us it simply means to strip the New Testament of the cultural trappings of the accepted male dominance and let Spirit, not sexual traditions, reign in our ecclesiastical organizations.

Spice Up Sex Life With Increased Ejaculation Volume

Many men are thinking about improving their performance in bed with an increased ejaculation volume. Increasing the sperm volume is not as hard as it seems, and it can be done easily. Plenty of men are seeking methods on how to increase cum volume, and they have been doing it more over the last few years.

Sperm production means you can release with more power increase the semen volume and raise the fertility rate as well as sperm count. There are many sperm pills that are available to do the needful. However these are better option than foods. There are foods that can be taken but the sex pills will have more effect than the foods.

To increase the seminal flow however men have to understand what it is before they get involved with the production. There is a natural process, by abstaining from sexual activity for a long time. If the sexual activity is controlled for at least one to three weeks, there will be a good increase in the sperm count. This will also help with greater ejaculation.

Many men do not prefer this method because they have to abstain from sexual activity. Heat will surely reduce sperm production, so the kind of clothes that are worn should be kept in check. A good diet is very important when it comes to increasing ejaculation volume. Those men with this problem must also make sure that they drink a lot of water and keep the body hydrated well.

Vitamins are also a good choice that can be taken every day, and then the sperm supplements can also be taken. If taken these cum pills then it should be all natural products, as you would not want any complications. There should be a healthy number of sperms while ejaculating once, and it should be kept at this level.

This disorder is mainly caused because most men today are faced with stress. Not only, that they also consume a lot of alcohol and smoke as well. Because of the stress they will be consuming less food too. Once all these factors are controlled, there will not be many complaints about the fertility. There seem to be a growing number of men reporting a drop in fertility rates.

All this can be avoided with a healthy lifestyle and if need be one can also consume sex pills for a better sperm production.

Some Important Facts about Vibrators

Vibrator is as an electrical and mainly battery operated device. Therere also all-mains vibrators. Their main quality is vibration. When placed against some erogenous zone it causes intensive and very pleasant sensations. Majority of people fancy vibrator as a penis-shaped object, yet such an opinion erroneous, since therere vibrators of various shapes and sizes and, as a rule, they arent meant for penetration. Upon usage the tip of vibrator is placed against highly sensitive erogenous zone. Vibrators can be purchased at drugstores, sex shops and female underwear shops.

Vibrator is the right instrument to break female self-conceit and assurance in that she can control her emotions in any situation. Sexual stimulation with the help of vibrator is so intense that its almost impossible to resist it. Vibrator can bring a woman to orgasm in case she had never experienced it before. Having once experienced strong effect of vibrator henceforth a woman will get many opportunities to achieve orgasm independently or with a partner.

Thus, vibrator can be used by a woman for self-stimulation. Sometimes her partner can use vibrator to stimulate female erogenous zones upon her desires. Vibrator can also be used for male sexual stimulation, yet vibrating effect on males is less effective than on females. At the same time men also have erogenous zones that can react violently to vibration. Theyre located on the back of penis and in the area between scrotum and anus.

Its recommended to be fastidious while choosing vibrator. Youd better buy a vibrator produced by some well-known company. Your vibrator should always be clean. For example, if you use your vibrator in anal region, then, before moving it to your vagina or any other place, wash the vibrator thoroughly. Remember that if you use your vibrator for sexual stimulation of genitals of both partners, it can become a source of sexually transmitted infectious diseases.

And another warning: vibrator gives us huge possibilities; nevertheless its influence can become really tyrannical. In other words long and intensive vibrator usage may lead to dependence and any other ways of sexual stimulation will become ineffective. As a result it would be very difficult for your partner to stimulate you. Thats why if youre going to lead healthy and versatile sexual life with your present or future partner, dont be much carried away with vibrators in order to keep the ability to orgasm with other means of sexual stimulation.

Size Matters More to Men

Sigmund Freud, the father of Psychiatry, said that men had a sexual thought consciously or subconsciously every 3 seconds. He timed it like a racehorse when he wasnt busy having sexual relations with his mother. Psychiatrists go to school for 22 years, subject themselves to years of Psychotherapy, then sit while you ramble and beg for advice for 45 minutes, only to say at the end, What do you think? Im afraid our time is up for this week. You could go insane merely from their torture tactics.

Obviously penis size matters to a woman. Penises range in size from 1 to 14 on men. The longer and wider and harder the penis, the more friction is created, the deeper the penetration, and the more likely the woman is to achieve vaginal orgasm. However other things are more important to a woman, such as extended foreplay, clitoral stimulation to orgasm, g spot stimulation to orgasm, and length of time after intercourse before the man hails a cab, generally anywhere from 5 to 7 minutes on average.

Size definitely matters to women, but it matters far more to men. Penis envy is not a female phenomenon despite the ravings of the incestuous Dr. Freud. Penis envy is a male phenomenon. Envying the length and width of the black penis is at the root of the Klu Klux Klan, says Mariah Carey. According to research done at Heidelberg University, it is a scientific fact that the purchases of Corvettes and BMWs are inversely proportional to the length of a mans penis. Men think that if they have an expensive fancy car then women will think that they are financially successful and will date them, leading other men to think that they are stacked.

The basic theme of any male Rap song and video is always the same. I am the coolest most hung baddest dude in town and I can ride you all night long. This is always backed up by half naked stunning harem women slithering around the artist. The lack of a white boxing champion for the past 75 years since Rocky Marciano, has led white men to flock to seven sequels of the Rocky movie. Rocky is now coming out of retirement, the Italian Stallion, for a rematch against Kanye West, who has been paid 5 million dollars to take a dive in the fifth, to soothe the wounded egos of male White America, and thats what its all about anyway, Ego.

The Ego is the part of the brain that either says in your mind, I am wonderful, or I am garbage. The Id is the part of your brain that says I want food, water, sex etc. The Ego is what causes men to desire multiple partners endlessly through cyber dating, because once a woman gives in, no matter how beautiful she is, no matter how loving and caring, she has now lost the ability to give to the man the thing he wants most to boost his Ego, that initial conquest, that triggers in the mans mind, I am great, I conquered her. Men need this to compensate for wounded Egos received at the hands of their insecure fathers, because criticism and control make the father feel great, to compensate for their own reality, unfulfilled wives due to their tiny narrow limp phallus. This is the root cause of the male mid life crisis, leading to divorce and insecure offspring because the male now needs a young wife the same way that he needs a Corvette. Have you ever noticed the shape of a Corvette?

This would all be bad enough but size issues are at the root of male competitiveness in both sports and war. Kim Jong Il, the mini me leader of North Korea has a stable of gorgeous young blonde American women, to make up for his tiny thang. Thats all you got, baby? Those words led to the swift execution of a one hit wonder American Diva who was all into the Grace Kelly thing. This would be bad enough, but the development of nuclear weapons and the verbal bravado of this midget against the United States is directly linked to the madman midgets size insecurity. Ironically midgets are generally very well endowed in proportion to their body size, and this is why they have such confidence. A well known self confidence building mantra used extensively by the Moonies, is My rooster is huge and hard, and I can ride you all night long. The problem has become so bad, that erectile dysfunction has become the third leading growth industry worldwide, and men are running for medication named after the enormous gushing of the massive powerful power generating Niagara Falls, even knowing that it causes a rare but pervasive form of blindness.

Martha Stewart has a solution for this insecurity problem which is now leading us all into the Apocalypse, the sudden violent end of all life on Earth forever. The Christian people are eagerly constructing and waiting for the Apocalypse, so that when it comes, after about 30 seconds, they can all say as One, Look, we were right! This need to be right, and this unbearable pain of being wrong, is a direct result of penis insecurity. Martha's solution is that all men be forced to wear their bag and their bone on their foreheads, for all to see, to instantly put an end to all the b/s and bluffing leading us all into the nuclear inferno. Oprah seconds the motion. She has the most to lose, according to Dr. Phil, the bald barking know it all with the 3 inch penis. Our modern Dr. Freud wears a sock folded in his pants to hide his shortcomings. Maybe an international naked at work day is the answer for saving life on earth. Maybe the Apocalypse wont be that bad. At least it will put an end to the zillions of Erectile Dysfunction (medications for 1 inch shriveled up things that refuse to stand up no matter how much kiddy porn the man watches) emails in our email boxes. How do these snake oil salesmen get our addresses anyways? Why arent they all blind yet? The insecurity disease has now spread to women rushing for breast implants, and to the male obsession with increasing their Google Page Ranking. Have you ever noticed the graphic that Sergey Brin and Larry Page use to display that ranking? They didnt become zillionaires at 32 by being oblivious to the male fixation with size now, did they?

J'aime le sexe

www.ingramcontent.com/pod-product-compliance
Lightning Source LLC
Chambersburg PA
CBHW031124160726

47989CB00016B/1007